HARVARD MEDICAL SCHOOL

BRIGHAM and WOMEN'S HOSPITAL

NORMAN K. HOLLENBERG, M.D., Ph.D.
(617) 732-6682   734-3349

75 FRANCIS STREET
BOSTON, MASSACHUSETTS 02115

Dear Colleague:

The management of hypertension has undergone significant evolution over the past two decades. There has been a trend toward the treatment of milder hypertension, and hypertension in the older individual, based upon impressive scientific evidence to indicate that treatment begets benefit. At the same time, the range of effective and well-tolerated antihypertensive agents has increased. A third element has involved the increasing recognition that the pathogenesis of coronary artery disease, the major residual cause of morbidity and mortality in the patient treated for hypertension, is multifactorial, and that changing the natural history of coronary artery disease in the hypertensive patient will require an approach based on that recognition. Hence, the structure of this book.

To assist in the application to daily practice of this information, "Management of Hypertension: A Multifactorial Approach" has been written. The authors and I are pleased that E.R. Squibb & Sons has had the insight to make this book available to practitioners, and are hopeful that you will find the information useful in designing treatment for your patients with hypertension.

Sincerely,

Norman K. Hollenberg, M.D., Ph.D.
Director & Professor

Management of Hypertension:

A Multifactorial Approach

Norman K. Hollenberg, MD, PhD
Editor

Scientific Therapeutics Information, Inc

Butterworths

Boston □ London □ Singapore □ Sydney □ Toronto □ Wellington

MANAGEMENT OF HYPERTENSION: A MULTIFACTORIAL APPROACH

Norman K. Hollenberg, MD, PhD

This book has been prepared by independent authors. E.R. Squibb & Sons assumes no responsibility either for the contents or for the judgments contained herein. Before prescribing any Squibb products mentioned, please refer to the full prescribing information provided at the end of the text.

Captopril may be used as initial therapy in hypertension only for patients with normal renal function in whom the risk of neutropenia/agranulocytosis is relatively low (1 out of over 8,600 in clinical trials). Captopril is indicated in patients with heart failure who have not responded adequately to or cannot be controlled by conventional diuretic and digitalis therapy; it is to be used with diuretics and digitalis. Use special precautions in patients with impaired renal function, collagen vascular disorders, or those exposed to other drugs known to affect the white cells or immune response. Evaluation of patients should always include assessment of renal function. See INDICATIONS AND USAGE, WARNINGS, and ADVERSE REACTIONS in the full prescribing information on the last pages.

Printed in the United States of America

First printing

First edition

Library of Congress Cataloging in Publication Data

Management of Hypertension: A Multifactorial Approach

Includes bibliography and index.
1. Hypertension
   Hollenberg, Norman K.

   ISBN 0-936871-04-0

Scientific Therapeutics Information, Inc
505 Morris Avenue
Springfield, NJ 07081

Table of Contents

Contributors

David B. Case, MD
Clinical Associate Professor of Medicine
Department of Medicine
Cornell University Medical College
New York, New York

Robert S. Eliot, MD, FACC
Director
Cardiovascular Institute
Swedish Medical Center
Denver, Colorado

William F. Graettinger, MD
Assistant Professor of Medicine
Veterans Administration Medical Center
Long Beach, California

Norman K. Hollenberg, MD, PhD
Director and Professor of Physiologic
   Research
Departments of Radiology and Medicine
Harvard Medical School
Brigham and Women's Hospital
Boston, Massachusetts

Norman M. Kaplan, MD
Professor of Medicine
Department of Internal Medicine
University of Texas Health Science Center
Dallas, Texas

Barry J. Materson, MD
Professor of Medicine
University of Miami
Veterans Administration Medical Center
Miami, Florida

Hugo M. Morales-Ballejo, MD, FACC
Director of Clinical Research
Cardiovascular Institute
Swedish Medical Center
Denver, Colorado

Leopoldo Raij, MD
Chief, Nephrology/Hypertension
Veterans Administration Medical Center
Professor of Medicine
University of Minnesota Medical School
Minneapolis, Minnesota

Marcia A. Testa, MPh, PhD
Senior Lecturer
Department of Biostatistics
Harvard School of Public Health
Boston, Massachusetts

Jonathan P. Tolins, MD
Veterans Administration Medical Center
Assistant Professor of Medicine
University of Minnesota School of Medicine
Minneapolis, Minnesota

Michael A. Weber, MD
Professor of Medicine
Hypertension Center
Veterans Administration Medical Center
Long Beach, California

Gordon A. Williams, MD
Chief, Endocrinology-Hypertension Service
Professor of Medicine
Brigham and Women's Hospital
Boston, Massachusetts

Preface

Norman K. Hollenberg, MD, PhD

As recently as 1966, thoughtful physicians with a strong interest in the problem of hypertension were able to maintain an "attitude of skepticism and restraint in accepting drugs that lower blood pressure as even a partial answer to the management of hypertensive disease" (Goldring and Chasis, 1966). One year later, the first report from the Veterans Administration Cooperative Study Group (1967) made it clear that drug treatment indeed reduced the morbidity of hypertension, at least in patients with a diastolic blood pressure over 115 mm Hg.

These findings prompted a revolution in therapeutics. A major focus of this revolution has been the importance of attempts to alter the natural history of chronic processes. No better example exists than the treatment of hypertension, where a series of carefully controlled trials has made it clear that treatment is worthwhile (Amery et al, 1985; Helgeland, 1980; Hypertension Detection and Follow-up Program [HDFP] Cooperative Group, 1979a; Medical Research Council [MRC] Working Party, 1985; Multiple Risk Factor Intervention Trial Research Group, 1982; Report by the Management Committee, 1980; Smith, 1977; Veterans Administration [VA] Cooperative Study Group, 1967, 1970).

Our major problem in the treatment of hypertension is that we do not provide symptom relief; rather, our goal is a change in natural history. Treatment that has as its goal a change in natural history, without providing symptom relief, is fundamentally more difficult because of the compliance problem (Haynes et al, 1982). Obviously, symptom relief provides a spur to compliance, but there are no symptoms directly related to hypertension. The problem grows even more difficult as we try to treat mild hypertension, where the goal of changing natural history is clearly long term and the spur to compliance is even more limited.

There has also been a continuing evolution in the drugs available for treatment and in recommendation concerning therapy—who to treat (Freis, 1982; Hollenberg, 1982; Kaplan, 1982; Laragh, 1982; Moser, 1982) and how to treat (Kaplan and Lieberman, 1982). Not surprisingly, that has been accompanied by an evolution in our expectations. The physician demands reliable evidence (for example, that a therapeutic agent is effective, provides predictable results, and is sufficiently well tolerated) that the patient will stay on treatment. Patients, aware of the enormous advances that medicine has made, expect treatment to be effective and to provide minimal or no side effects. Expectations of regulatory agencies reflect the needs of both the physicians and the patients. As a result, a wide variety of efficacious and safe regimens are now available from which to select.

Specificity of an agent in reversing a mechanism that is disordered is another general goal of antihypertensive therapy, and we would like to choose our agents on that basis. Unfortunately, we know too little about the pathogenesis of hypertension to make that ideal a factor in selecting an agent for an individual patient.

The frequency and nature of the low-grade side effects that can plague a patient and lead to discontinuation of treatment must be criteria for drug selection. Until this time, our focus in identifying the adverse reactions to an agent has involved physical manifestations, such as rash, gastrointestinal upset, or fatigue. When an agent impacted on a patient's emotional status or intellectual function, it was recognized only when the impact was sufficiently extreme to be obvious. To a major degree, the evolution of therapy for hypertension reflects a progressive improvement in this latter aspect of the drug profile, especially for agents used in place of, or in addition to, thiazide diuretics. Only the more "mature" physicians remember when patients were treated with a ganglionic blocking agent: patients were often normotensive but were severely constipated, impotent, and frequently had severe postural hypotension leading to dizziness and syncope. Reserpine was easier to use but because of the doses required, patients were extraordinarily sleepy and often depressed to the point of suicide. The advent of methyldopa and then propranolol and newer β-blockers improved therapy at each step because the low-grade central nervous system side effects that led to depression and fatigue became less frequent than with reserpine. However, as reviewed below, the frequency of these untoward effects is still substantial with these agents.

In our attempt to treat a large number of patients with milder hypertension and keep them in therapy, it is easy to predict that quality of life will become an increasingly important consideration. Despite the debate regarding at what level of blood pressure treatment should be initiated, we will be treating milder hypertension. Fortunately, substantial consideration has been given to the methodologic issues involved in assessing quality of life (Bulpitt et al, 1976; Garfield et al, 1976; Lloyd, 1983), as addressed by Dr. Marcia A. Testa and Dr. Gordon A. Williams in Chapter V.

Hypertension does not produce symptoms unless severe, but our patients with hypertension often have more symptoms than a normotensive comparison group, even when the hypertension is not being treated with drugs (Bulpitt et al, 1976).

Studies unrelated to hypertension have taught us a great deal that is relevant. One report suggested that 12% of patients in a family practice are likely to be the "worried well" (Garfield et al, 1976), a figure that seems low to me. Lloyd (1983) analyzed a number of data bases and suggested that 38% of patients in internal medicine practice are likely to have no demonstrable pathology to account for symptoms. Symptoms in an apparently healthy sample of the population are common (Reidenberg and Lowenthal, 1968).

Perhaps the increased frequency of symptoms in the hypertensive population represents a form of ascertainment bias. When individuals with a variety of complaints find their way into the health care system, one of three things can happen. One possibility is that the cause of the complaint will be identified and treated—a happy outcome. Another possibility is that the patients are found to have no demonstrable organic pathology to account for their symptoms. A third possibility is that no proven pathology can be found to account for the symptoms but high blood pressure *is* found. The patients are then labeled hypertensive and receive evaluation and care for that problem. They are left, however, with their original symptoms and the anxiety and depression that might have been responsible for the symptoms in the first place.

The available data are consonant with this view. In the classic study of Bulpitt et al (1976), the frequency of frank depression in the labeled but as yet untreated hypertensives in the six months covered by the study was an extraordinary 44.7%. Untreated hypertensives also suffered more frequently from nocturia, impotence, weakness, fatigue, and "slow walking pace," all of which are common physical expressions of anxiety or depression. Indeed, most practitioners would suspect that anxiety and depression are the most common cause of these physical complaints. Symptoms, thus, could be found with much greater frequency in hypertensives, although unrelated to the hypertension. They reflect the reason that the hypertension was identified in the first place.

The clinical situation is confounded further by the impact of "labeling," that is, being converted from a "person" to a "patient" with hypertension. At this juncture, individuals may well change their perceptions of themselves and their lifestyles. For example, the frequency of absenteeism rose strikingly after individuals were labeled hypertensive (Haynes et al, 1978).

Once therapy is initiated, the frequency of complaints rises sharply (Bulpitt and Dollery, 1973; Bulpitt et al, 1976; Curb et al, 1985a; Jachuck et al, 1982; MRC Working Party, 1981). Indeed, the frequency of complaints elicited from the patients under treatment may underestimate the magnitude of the problem (Jachuck et al, 1982).

Interest in sexual impairment has often focused on impotence (Stevenson and Umstead, 1984), presumably because it provides an unequivocal endpoint. A sharp reduction in libido is more common and occurs in women as frequently as in men. These observations probably account for the large number of patients who drop out of therapy (Curb et al, 1985a; MRC Working Party, 1981).

Do the findings on withdrawal from treatment in these reports reflect what happens in practice? The withdrawal rates, 20% or higher in both studies, underestimate the magnitude of the problem. Each study represented an enormous investment, and success was prejudiced by patient withdrawal. Substantial resources were made available to keep patients in treatment. In the practice setting, such resources are not available, and many more patients are likely to withdraw. Indeed, only 20% to 30% of individuals who know themselves to be hypertensive are under adequate blood pressure control (Haynes et al, 1982).

This book focuses on converting enzyme inhibition in the patient with hypertension. It is instructive to compare the withdrawal rates from large-scale studies employing angiotensin-converting enzyme inhibitors. In an analysis of 5679 patients with moderate and severe hypertension from a large number of trials, the dropout rate on captopril was about 6% (Jenkins et al, 1985). In smaller, multicenter trials involving several hundred patients treated with captopril, the dropout rate was substantially less than 5% in each case (Drayer and Weber, 1983; Kaneko et al, 1982; VA Cooperative Study Group, 1984; Weinberger, 1985), but the trials were substantially shorter than the MRC and HDFP trials mentioned above (Curb et al, 1985a; MRC Working Party, 1981). Reported dropouts on enalapril have also been low (Smith, 1984).

Comparisons of withdrawal rates from trials that differ in selection for entry and duration of therapy may be misleading. The dropout rate may be sensitive to patient education, to the setting of the trial, to preconceptions of the investigators, or to a host of uncontrolled factors. What of dropout rates in trials in which captopril was compared with alternative agents? In one double-blind trial (Kaneko et al, 1982), captopril was employed in 157 patients and propranolol in 167. The dropout rate on propranolol was four times higher than withdrawal from treatment with captopril. Similarly, when captopril was compared to either methyldopa or propranolol in several hundred patients on a double-blind basis, the withdrawal rate for captopril was about 6%, as opposed to 14% for propranolol and 20% for methyldopa (Croog et al, 1986).

It is interesting to note the use of antidepressants in patients treated with antihypertensive therapy that interacts with the central nervous system. Before a physician will prescribe a tricyclic antidepressant, he or she must be convinced that depression is sufficiently severe to justify such potent and potentially toxic agents. Tricyclic antidepressant use was significantly higher in patients taking β-blockers (23%) than for patients taking hydralazine or hypoglycemic agents (both 15%), agents not thought to impact on the central nervous system (Avorn et al, 1986). Perhaps equally surprising was the finding that methyldopa or reserpine showed a rather lower frequency ($\sim$10%) given their well-documented influence in promoting depression. Perhaps the answer lies in biases created by the fact that their influence on the central nervous system is widely known. An individual treated with methyldopa or reserpine who develops depression is more likely to have the antihypertensive discontinued than to have a tricyclic antidepressant added to the regimen.

The modern era of antihypertensive therapy has been a great success as study after study has documented the efficacy of therapy in an increasingly milder stage or form of the process. On the other hand, we have new challenges. One challenge involves the frequency of poor adherence to therapy and frank dropouts from treatment. If compliance is a problem in the treatment of a chronic, painful, and progressively disabling disease such as rheumatoid arthritis—and it often is (Katz, 1982)—the problem of compliance in hypertension treatment is substantially more difficult. Several chapters in this book will address this issue through approaches based on individualization of treatment and on quality of life considerations.

Our second challenge involves changing the natural history of atherosclerotic disease in the patient with hypertension. Controlled trials on the treatment of hypertension have made it clear that complications that can be considered "biophysical" in origin, such as stroke, heart failure, renal failure, encephalopathy, and dissecting aneurysm, become rare with effective treatment (Amery et al, 1985; HDFP Cooperative Group, 1979a; Helgeland, 1980; MRC Working Party, 1985; Report by the Management Committee, 1980; Smith, 1977; VA Cooperative Study Group, 1967, 1970). Antihypertensive therapy was essentially ineffective in reducing the frequency of atherosclerosis-related complications. One possible exception was the MRC report (1985) where propranolol may have reduced the frequency of myocardial infarction in a subgroup identified post hoc. If the post hoc analysis is accepted, the positive influence of propranolol was restricted to males who did not smoke and not to females or to male smokers. Even if present, the effect was small. A second exception was the European Working Party Trial of hypertension treatment in the elderly (Amery et al, 1985). This study, the first to address the problem of thiazide-induced electrolyte disarray by employing a potassium-sparing combination in a controlled trial, was also the first to document a clear reduction in death both from heart disease and from myocardial infarction, although the frequency of occurrence was not reduced. In planning treatment with thiazide diuretics (and they are frequently required), we must be aware of the importance of the electrolyte disarray that they induce. Our choice is a potassium-sparing combination or a converting-enzyme inhibitor.

An important lesson that has emerged from epidemiological studies is the interaction between risk factors for atherosclerosis. The increase in risk to an individual in being a heavy smoker, having high blood pressure, and an increase in serum cholesterol is much more than the sum of the individual risks. Based on the premise that we will have to deal with each source of risk in such patients to prevent the progression of atherosclerosis, substantial attention has been given to the risk factors for atherosclerosis in the chapters that follow.

There are few branches of medicine in which physicians do not often encounter the patient with hypertension. This book was organized and written with that fact in mind.

Chapter I

Perspectives on Contemporary Management of Hypertension

Barry J. Materson, MD

INTRODUCTION

Hypertension is a disorder of arterial pressure regulation characterized by cardiovascular pathologic changes proportionate to the degree and duration of arterial pressure elevation. This definition ties together the following concepts:

- Hypertension is a disorder of regulatory mechanism(s).
- Hypertension will cause abnormalities of the heart and vascular system. All other target organ damage is a function of vascular pathology.
- The damage is a product of the quantities of pressure elevation and time. Severe hypertension will effect pathological abnormalities within months to a few years. Placebo-controlled trials are no longer ethical tests of treatment modalities for severe hypertension. In contrast, very mild hypertension may require decades in order to achieve measurable endpoints. Large-scale, long-term epidemiological trials (ideally placebo controlled) are required to demonstrate the benefit of a given intervention.

In order to focus on the concept, this definition omits specific quantifiers that are necessary for employers, insurance companies, the military, clinical investigators, and the practicing physician. Numerical limits are needed to guide the approach. These limits are useful so long as we appreciate that they are arbitrary and not indicative of the biological continuum of hypertension. Tables I and II are the recommendations of the Joint National Committee on Detection, Evaluation, and Treatment of High Blood Pressure (The Joint National Committee, 1984). These are carefully thought out and translate definition to action.

We have come a long way in our understanding of hypertension and in our ability to treat it effectively. Review of Table III provides an interesting perspective of the chronology of therapy for hypertension. None of the therapeutic modalities introduced prior to 1949 has remained in use after 1960. The three basic drugs that made modern therapy of hypertension possible were

---

Table I.   **Classification of blood pressure (from the Joint National Committee, 1984, with permission).**

Range, mm Hg	Category[a]
Diastolic	
<85	Normal blood pressure
85–89	High-normal blood pressure
90–104	Mild hypertension
105–114	Moderate hypertension
≥115	Severe hypertension
Systolic, when diastolic blood pressure is <90	
<140	Normal blood pressure
140–159	Borderline isolated systolic hypertension
≥160	Isolated systolic hypertension

[a]A classification of borderline isolated systolic hypertension (SBP, 140 mm Hg to 159 mm Hg) or isolated systolic hypertension (SBP, >160 mm Hg) takes precedence over a classification of high-normal blood pressure (DBP, 85 mm Hg to 89 mm Hg) when both occur in the same person. A classification of high-normal blood pressure (DBP, 85 mm Hg to 89 mm Hg) takes precedence over a classification of normal blood pressure (SBP, <140 mm Hg) when both occur in the same person.

---

introduced into use between 1953 and 1958 (rauwolfia, 1953; hydralazine, 1953; thiazide diuretics, 1958), with the thiazides enabling the use of reserpine and hydralazine in "nontoxic" doses. In the past decade alone, the list of available drugs has doubled. The availability of the angiotensin-converting enzyme inhibitors has helped change the philosophy of treatment of hypertension to one of not simply lowering the blood pressure toward normal but doing so with a minimal perturbation of the patient's quality of life.

We now appreciate that essential hypertension is not a homogenous entity and that its multifactorial nature requires a multipronged approach. Nondrug as well as pharmacologic therapy has achieved recognition as have other controllable environmental factors. None of us has yet found a way to select his or her own parents with a view toward getting a better genetic composition. We are, however, learning to deal with those adverse environmental factors that unmask the genetic expression of hypertension in those who have a genetic predisposition.

This chapter points out the benefits of lowering blood pressure using data from major epidemiologic trials, addresses the controversy on the limited effects of blood pressure reduction on coronary heart disease, reviews the basic philosophy of nondrug and pharmacological therapy, discusses the issue of quality of life, and reviews some of the past, present, and perhaps future strategies for drug therapy of hypertension.

BENEFITS OF LOWERING BLOOD PRESSURE

Mild Hypertension That hypertension is associated with increased risk of coronary heart disease, intermittent claudication, stroke, congestive heart failure, and death was not at all controversial in 1987. What is very much an issue is drug therapy of the largest group of hypertensive patients, those with diastolic

---

Table II.   **Follow-up criteria (from the Joint National Committee, 1984, with permission).**

Range, mm Hg	Recommended follow-up[a]

Follow-up Criteria for First-occasion Measurement

Diastolic

<85	Recheck within 2 years
85–89	Recheck within 1 year
90–104	Confirm promptly (not to exceed 2 months)
105–114	Evaluate or refer promptly to source of care (not to exceed 2 weeks)
≥115	Evaluate or refer immediately to a source of care

Systolic, when diastolic blood pressure is <90

<140	Recheck within 2 years
140–199	Confirm promptly (not to exceed 2 months)
≥200	Evaluate or refer promptly to source of care (not to exceed 2 weeks)

Follow-up Criteria for Second-occasion Measurement

Diastolic

<85	Recheck within 2 years[b]
85–89	Recheck within 1 year
≥90	Evaluate or refer promptly to a source of care

Systolic, when diastolic blood pressure is <90

<140	Recheck within 1 year
≥140	Evaluate or refer promptly to a source of care

---

[a] If recommendations for follow-up of diastolic and systolic blood pressure are different for those aged 18 years or older, the shorter recommended time period supersedes and a referral supersedes a recheck recommendation.

[b] Rechecking within one year is recommended for persons at increased risk of progressing to higher blood pressure, including family history of hypertension or cardiovascular event, weight gain or obesity, black race, use of an oral contraceptive, and excessive ethanol consumption.

blood pressure 90 mm Hg to 104 mm Hg. They tend to be asymptomatic, have the least immediate benefit of treatment, and are likely to be the least tolerant of adverse effects of treatment. The point at which the benefits of treatment exceed the risks associated with drugs for the mildly hypertensive patient has not been clearly defined.

The implications of the argument are not trivial. Figure 1 displays the distribution of hypertensive patients at initial screening if hypertension is defined as a diastolic blood pressure ≥90 mm Hg. A change of the definition to ≥95 mm Hg would prevent 42.7% of that population from being labeled as hypertensive, and

Table III. **A chronology of therapy for essential hypertension (from Kaplan, 1986a, with permission).**

Modality	Year introduced	Time in use
Thiocyanate	1903	1925–1945
Low-salt diet	1904	1940–1960
Surgical sympathectomy	1925	1935–1960
Veratrum alkaloids	1940	1945–1950
Ganglionic blocking drugs	1947	1950–1955
Hydralazine	1949	1953
Rauwolfia	1949	1953
Thiazide diuretics	1957	1958
Spironolactone	1959	1960
Guanethidine	1959	1960
α-Methyldopa	1960	1962
MAO inhibitors	1960	1963–1970
Diazoxide	1962	1973
Furosemide	1964	1966
Propranolol[a]	1964	1976
Bethanidine	1964	1981
Debrisoquin[b]	1965	
Clonidine	1966	1975
Guancydine[b]	1969	
Guanadrel	1969	1983
Minoxidil	1970	1979
Prazosin	1972	1976
Guanabenz	1973	1983
Verapamil	1975	1986
Captopril	1977	1981
Labetalol	1977	1984
Nifedipine	1979	
Diltiazem	1981	
Enalapril	1981	1986

[a] A large number of β-adrenergic blockers have subsequently been introduced, and, as of March 1986, seven have been approved for use in the United States.
[b] These drugs have not been approved for use in the United States but are being used elsewhere.

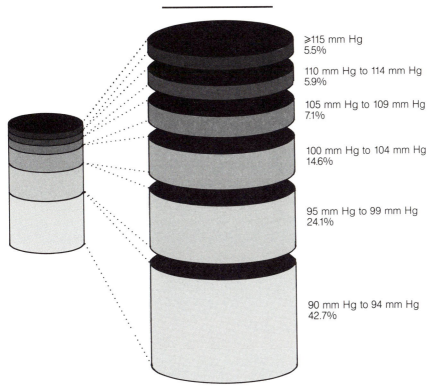

Figure 1.
Distribution of patients with varying degrees of diastolic
hypertension using diastolic blood pressure ≥90 mm Hg to define
hypertension. (Data were derived from Hypertension Detection and
Follow-up Program, 1977.)

they probably would not be exposed to drug therapy (Hypertension Detection and Follow-up Program [HDFP] Cooperative Group, 1977). Indeed, 81.4% of those initially screened for the HDFP were in the mildly hypertensive group (diastolic blood pressure 90 mm Hg to 104 mm Hg).

That initial screening found 25.3% of the target population to be hypertensive. On rescreening, only 14.5% had a diastolic blood pressure ≥90 mm Hg. After two rescreenings, the 10,940 hypertensive patients were distributed as follows: mild (90 mm Hg to 104 mm Hg), 71.5%; moderate (105 mm Hg to 114 mm Hg), 18.8%; and severe (≥115 mm Hg), 9.7% (HDFP Cooperative Group, 1979a). If one assumes that there were 26,542,000 Americans with hypertension in 1982 (Table IV), then about 19 million would have mild hypertension and approximately 10 million of those would be "mild-mild," with diastolic blood pressure 90 mm Hg to 94 mm Hg. The implications for cost of treatment, serious adverse effects (including possible promotion of atherosclerosis), and impact on quality of life are obvious. The key question then is: Does treatment of mild hypertension provide a meaningful benefit? The answer appears to be yes.

Changes in Death Rate   Table V displays the changes in crude death rate between 1960 and 1982 for selected cardiovascular diseases. Motor vehicle fatalities have been added as a frame of reference. Comparison of data from 1960 and 1982 reveals that major decrements in death rate have occurred with hypertensive heart disease (−72.2%), hypertension (−53.5%), cerebrovascular disease (−37%), and even ischemic heart disease (−19.7%). During the same period, all-cause mortality was declining by 10.7% and motor vehicle accident deaths by only 7%. Whether this decline in ischemic heart disease mortality is real is discussed thoroughly by Stern (1979). He pointed out that the approximate 20% decline in ischemic heart disease mortality was true of all age groups, both sexes, and the three major racial/ethnic groups. His review indicated that these decreases were not simply an artifact of changing the way cause of death is reported on death

---

Table IV.   **Characteristics of the hypertensive population.**[a]

Demographics	Rate per 1000 persons	Number of persons
Overall	116.9	26,542,000
Male	101.3	11,411,000
Female	131.4	15,660,000
Age <18 years	2.9	182,400
18–44 years	58.9	5,775,000
45–64 years	245.7	10,950,000
Over 65 years	390.4	10,490,000

[a] Data for 1982 derived from Tables 25, 27, and 187 (US Bureau of the Census, 1985). Derived numbers have been rounded, and gender data were estimates for 1982. Therefore, the overall, gender, and age sums are somewhat different.

Table V.   **Crude death rate per 100,000 population for selected diseases from 1960 to 1982 (from US Bureau of the Census, 1985; Table 114).**

Disease	1960	1970	1980	1982
All causes	954.7	945.3	878.3	852.0
Major cardiovascular disease	515.1	496.0	436.4	417.6
Diseases of the heart	369.0	362.0	336.0	326.0
Hypertensive heart disease	37.0	7.4	10.9	10.3
Ischemic heart disease	296.9	328.1	249.7	238.5
Hypertension	7.1	4.1	3.5	3.3
Cerebrovascular disease	108.0	101.9	75.1	68.0
Atherosclerosis	20.0	15.6	13.0	11.6
Motor vehicle accidents	21.3	26.9	23.5	19.8

Table VI. **Effect of treatment on preventing progression from mild to more severe hypertension (diastolic blood pressure greater than 110 mm Hg): findings from major clinical trials (from Moser, 1986, with permission).**

| | Number of patients | | | |
| | Placebo | | Active treatment | |
Study (Range for mild hypertension)	Mild hyper-tension	Progressed to more severe disease	Mild hyper-tension	Progressed to more severe disease
US Public Health Cooperative Study (90 mm Hg to 114 mm Hg)	196	24[a]	193	0
Veterans Administration Cooperative Study (90 mm Hg to 114 mm Hg)	194	20	186	0
Australian Study (95 mm Hg to 109 mm Hg)	1,706	202	1,721	5
Oslo Study (90 mm Hg to 110 mm Hg)[b]	379	65	406	1
Medical Research Council Study (90 mm Hg to 109 mm Hg)	8,654	1,011	8,700	76
Total	11,129	1,318	11,206	82

[a] Diastolic blood pressure greater than 130 mm Hg.
[b] Systolic hypertension was present in only 12.5% of patients.

certificates. He suggested that the real reason for the decline was primary prevention. That is, favorable dietary changes, improved hypertension control, and other favorable changes in living habits made the major contribution to the decline.

Progression of Hypertension   Those who would view the gains of antihypertensive treatment of mild hypertensives as negligible generally do so by pointing out the large number of people who must be treated in order to prevent one cardiovascular death. Although this is true, this argument tends to ignore two important points. First, in major trials such as the HDFP, which did show a difference, the reference group was not a placebo group with uncontrolled hypertension but rather a treated group with blood pressure levels well within the acceptable goal of other trials. The second point is that in untreated groups or those less well treated, progression of hypertension and left ventricular hypertrophy continues while it is stopped or reversed in the treated group.

Table VI displays five major epidemiologic studies on mild to moderate hypertension that were placebo controlled. It is clear from these data that there is an enormous risk of progression to more severe disease in patients with mild to moderate hypertension who are left untreated. In fact, 11.8% (1318) of patients treated with placebo or no drug experienced progression of disease compared with only 0.7% (82) of the patients who received active treatment. Obviously, not all of these patients achieved goal blood pressure. It is, therefore, clear that even partially effective treatment is vastly superior to no treatment at all. The nature of these complications is shown in Table VII. Again, it is clear that a significant improvement was achieved in all categories, including coronary events, in the treated group.

The progression of hypertension has also been shown in adolescents. A group of 435 adolescents in Evans County, Georgia, were evaluated and followed in the 1960s. Using a systolic pressure ≥ 140 mm Hg and/or a diastolic pressure of ≥ 90 mm Hg as a definition, 11% had hypertension. Thirty patients from this group were followed for seven years, during which two died from hemorrhagic strokes. Three patients had sustained hypertension with cardiovascular and cerebrovascular symptoms. One developed hypertensive heart disease, and five more were found to have asymptomatic sustained hypertension. Interestingly, 12 became normotensive. Also of interest was the fact that four of the 30 controls developed hypertension over the period of observation. Obesity and subsequent further weight gain were impressive associated findings in the patients who developed sustained hypertension (Heyden et al, 1969).

Table VII.   Five therapeutic trials of mild hypertension: cumulative complications in control and treated groups[a] (from Moser, 1986, with permission).

Complications	Control		Treated		Percent improvement control-treated Control
	Number[b]	Percent	Number[b]	Percent	
Total morbid events	563	9.0	417	6.6	27
Total mortality	342	5.4	252	4.1	24
Cerebrovascular events:					
fatal and nonfatal	140	2.2	76	1.2	50
Fatal coronary events	79	1.2	46	0.7	42

[a] Data from the Veterans Administration Cooperative Study: diastolic blood pressure 90 mm Hg to 104 mm Hg; United States Public Health Cooperative Study Group; Hypertension Detection and Follow-up Program: Stratum 1; Australian Study; and Oslo Study.
[b] Total control and treated populations each comprise approximately 6400 subjects.

The Veterans Administration Trials Freis (1979) detailed the results of the Veterans Administration (VA) Cooperative Studies that proved unequivocally that treatment of moderate to severe hypertension reduced hypertensive complications. Although the data in support of treating mild hypertension were much less striking, there was strong indication that it would be of benefit in mild hypertension as well.

Public Health Service Trial The Public Health Service (Smith, 1977) studied 389 patients aged 21 to 55 with mild to moderate hypertension in a prospective, randomized, double-blind fashion. Patients were treated either with a combination of chlorothiazide 500 mg and rauwolfia serpentina 100 mg or placebo. Blood pressure was reduced by 16/10 mm Hg in the treatment group without change in the placebo group. Pathologic changes associated with hypertension, including electrocardiographic and radiologic evidence of left ventricular hypertrophy and hypertensive retinopathy, occurred in 15% of the drug-treated group compared with 33.2% of the placebo group. On the other hand, atherosclerotic changes, including myocardial infarction and other evidence of coronary heart disease, were approximately equal in the two groups: 14% of the actively treated group and 12.8% of the placebo group. There were two strokes in the placebo group and none in the active group. Adverse drug effects requiring termination occurred in only 5.9% of the cases.

Despite the fact that this group had demonstrated a 60% reduction in hypertensive complications, the investigators recommended systematic follow-up without drugs while attempting hygienic intervention and control of other risk factors. Further, they recommended that clinicians should consider delaying drug therapy in the mildly hypertensive group until evidence of electrocardiographic changes or a progressive rise in blood pressure was noted. Ten years later, this latter recommendation is not an acceptable strategy.

The Australian Trial The Australian therapeutic trial in mild hypertension is an exceedingly important study (Report by the Management Committee, 1980). The study group enrolled 3427 men and women with mild hypertension who were free from clinical evidence of cardiovascular disease. This is an important qualifier because almost all of the other studies admitted at least some patients who had prior evidence of atherosclerosis. For example, in the HDFP trial (HDFP Cooperative Group, 1979a), 5% of the patients had a history of myocardial infarction and 2% had a history of stroke. In addition, approximately 7% of patients were diabetics and 25% of patients were already receiving antihypertensive medications. The disadvantage of the Australian study was that it lasted only four years and dealt with patients with mild hypertension. Therefore, the rate of fatal and nonfatal trial endpoints was relatively low. Nevertheless, the difference in cumulative incidence of trial endpoints between the active and placebo groups for both fatal and nonfatal events was impressive and is displayed in Figure 2. There was a large reduction in cerebrovascular events in the actively treated group. The placebo group had double the number of fatal events, nearly double the number of nonfatal hemorrhagic or thrombotic strokes, and more than twice the number of transient ischemic attacks. Retinopathy occurred more frequently in the placebo group. Only three patients developed renal failure. One was on active treatment and two on placebo. Congestive heart failure occurred in

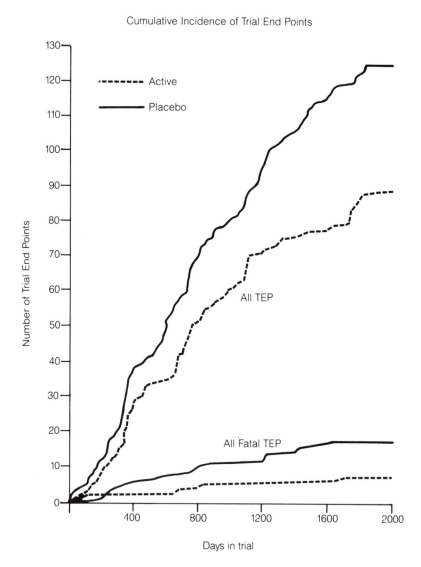

Cumulative Incidence of Trial End Points

Figure 2.
Cumulative occurrence of total trial endpoints (TEP) and of deaths from all causes in 1721 subjects of the active and 1706 of the placebo group while adhering to trial regimen. The difference between active and placebo groups was significant for all trial endpoints (p <0.01) and all deaths (p <0.05; from Report by the Management Committee, 1980, with permission).

only three patients. Two of those were receiving active treatment and one placebo.

It is sometimes said that this trial failed to show protection against ischemic heart disease, and that is true for nonfatal myocardial infarction and other nonfatal cardiac endpoints. On the other hand, there were two fatal ischemic cardiac events in the actively treated group compared with eight in the placebo group with the p value (p = 0.051) just missing the standard criterion for statistical significance. The study group estimated that if the rate of trial endpoints found in the patients participating in this study were applied to the general population of Australia, there would be on the average 7000 fewer episodes of cardiovascular disease per year, including about 2000 fewer strokes and 2000 fewer deaths per year.

Results of the Hypertension Detection and Follow-up Program Two years later, the HDFP Cooperative Group (1979a) published findings that brought tremendous pressure to bear on practicing physicians to treat even very mildly hypertensive patients. This multicenter group screened nearly 160,000 people and randomized 10,940 hypertensive patients to be treated either using a stepped-care protocol or referral to unstructured community medical therapy. At the time the study was designed, it was anticipated that the referred-care group would not be aggressively treated. The impact of the National Blood Pressure Education Program was greater than anticipated, however, and patients in the referred-care group were indeed treated, although not nearly as aggressively as those in the stepped-care group. The findings have had a major impact because they have encouraged physicians to treat even very mild hypertension. The results for the group with mild hypertension (90 mm Hg to 104 mm Hg) are of particular interest.

At the end of five years, approximately 75% of the stepped-care group were receiving medication, and 64% of patients in the group with mild hypertension were at or below blood pressure goal. This was in contrast to 54% of the referred-care group receiving treatment and 43% of these patients being at or below goal. Mean diastolic blood pressure was reduced by 12.9 mm Hg to 83.4 mm Hg in the stepped-care group and by 8.6 mm Hg to 87.8 mm Hg in the referred-care group. This net difference of 4.3 mm Hg at five years produced dramatic results. There was a 20.3% reduction in all-cause mortality, 26% fewer deaths from all cardiovascular diseases in the stepped-care group, and fewer deaths due to stroke and myocardial infarction. No differences were noted in death due to other ischemic heart disease or hypertensive heart disease.

When these data were analyzed for mortality by race, sex, and age (HDFP Cooperative Group, 1979b), the greatest benefits in regard to reduction in all-cause death rates occurred in white and black men and black women for the age subgroups 50 to 59 and 60 to 69 years. White women benefited least, but it was also this group that had the least difference between the stepped-care and referred-care group.

The mildly hypertensive group had 31.8% lower incidence of fatal and nonfatal stroke in the stepped-care group. The greatest protection against stroke was afforded those patients with severe hypertension and the group of patients aged 60 to 69 years (HDFP Cooperative Group, 1982). The conclusion of the HDFP Cooperative Group was "these findings support the premise that decreasing diastolic blood pressure reduces stroke morbidity and mortality in all those who have abnormal blood pressure elevations, regardless of race, sex, age, level of diastolic blood pressure elevation, or chronicity of the condition."

Hardy and Hawkins (1983) published a detailed and complex analysis of the results of the HDFP to determine whether improvements in mortality were directly related to the degree of blood pressure reduction prompted by the lack of a placebo control group in the program. They found a highly significant relationship between blood pressure, blood pressure goal, and medication status and the risk of subsequent mortality. With certain carefully detailed reservations, they concluded that the HDFP mortality results were consistent with findings in other studies in which a placebo control group was used, and this contributed additional evidence of efficacy for treatment of even mild hypertension.

In the HDFP trial, only 8.6% of the mild hypertensives had definite or probable drug-related side effects. Hospitalization was required for less than 1% of all the active participants because of adverse effects. Sexual dysfunction required discontinuation in 8.3% of the men in the study. Overall, treatment was deemed to be relatively safe (Curb et al, 1985a).

Results of the Multiple Risk Factor Intervention Trial   Just as the HDFP data were beginning to have an impact, a potentially contrary signal emerged from the Multiple Risk Factor Intervention Trial (MRFIT; 1982). The goal of this study was to determine the benefit of reducing cardiovascular risk factors on the incidence of cardiovascular mortality. In this trial, a special intervention (SI) group that received intensive risk factor reduction therapy and a community-based usual care (UC) group as a control were used in a fashion analogous to the stepped-care and referred-care control group of HDFP. Unfortunately, the data in this trial were seriously confounded by the success in risk factor reduction achieved in the control group. In addition, approximately 4.5% of the total study population had major electrocardiographic (ECG) abnormalities and about 28% had a combination of major or minor ECG abnormalities on entry. Approximately 12% had ischemic responses to exercise. Subgroup analysis was performed for the patients with and without resting ECG abnormalities. In those patients who were normotensive, there was a somewhat (but not statistically significant) greater mortality in the UC group both in the absence and presence of resting ECG abnormalities. It is important to note that the mortality rate per thousand was 25.7 for the UC group versus 18.6 for the SI group when ECG abnormalities were present, even in the absence of hypertension. Hypertensive patients without ECG abnormalities had 20.7 per 1000 deaths due to coronary heart disease in the UC group versus 15.8 in the SI group. Confusion arises from those hypertensive patients with resting ECG abnormalities. In these patients, the SI group experienced 29.2 per 1000 deaths due to coronary heart disease, with 17.7 in the UC group. These data have been interpreted to suggest that the more aggressive intervention in the SI group, particularly with regard to thiazide diuretics, increased the risk for death related to coronary heart disease in that subset of patients who were hypertensive and had ECG abnormalities at baseline. The implication is that the diuretic treatment itself was responsible for the increased mortality (MRFIT, 1985).

In order to determine the influence of diuretic therapy on mortality, the Oslo study group reanalyzed their results according to the criteria used in MRFIT. Although the number of events was very small and did not achieve statistical significance, there was a somewhat higher incidence of coronary heart disease events in the group that was treated with hydrochlorothiazide (Holme et al, 1984).

Results of the Medical Research Council Trial   The Medical Research Council (MRC) Working Party (1985) began a single-blind, prospective trial of the treatment of mild hypertension in 1977. They recruited 17,354 patients with a diastolic blood pressure of 90 mm Hg to 109 mm Hg and aged 35 to 64 years. Patients were randomly assigned to treatment with either bendrofluazide, propranolol, or placebo. The results of this trial confirmed that active treatment reduced the incidence of stroke and all cardiovascular events. However, no difference was apparent in the overall rates of coronary events or all-cause mortality. One of the most fascinating aspects of the trial was the subgroup analyses. The authors were very cautious in their presentation and interpretation of these data because post hoc subgroup analyses are much less statistically powerful than analysis of the primary questions. Nevertheless, an exceedingly important negative impact of smoking was observed, particularly in patients who received propranolol. In the subgroup analyses, men receiving active treatment had a significantly lower all-cause mortality than men on placebo, but women actually had a slight increase with active treatment. The reduction in stroke rate was much greater in patients who were treated with diuretic than those who were treated with propranolol. Bendrofluazide did lower the stroke rate in both smokers and nonsmokers, but propranolol had no beneficial effect in the smokers. On the other hand, the rate of coronary events was not influenced by treatment with diuretic in either smokers or nonsmokers or in smokers treated with propranolol. However, propranolol was effective in reducing the coronary event rate in nonsmokers. This same pattern was observed for the rate of all cardiovascular events. The data for stroke are displayed in Figure 3 and those for coronary events in Figure 4.

Mild Hypertension in the Elderly   The European Working Party on High Blood Pressure in the Elderly (EWPHE) trial provided long-awaited information on whether treatment benefited patients with mild to moderate hypertension above age 60 (Amery et al, 1985). Prior to this study, there was only a suggestion that patients above age 60 may benefit from treatment. However, prior trials did not contain adequate numbers of patients in the 60 and above group to achieve statistical significance even though treatment had a favorable effect. For example, the VA Cooperative Study Group trial (1972) showed a 59% reduction in cardiovascular terminating versus nonterminating events in patients aged 60 or older and the Australian trial showed a reduction of 39% (Report by the Management Committee, 1980). These results are comparable with the 36% reduction that was statistically significant in the EWPHE trial. This very carefully performed double-blind, randomized, placebo-controlled study used hydrochlorothiazide plus triamterene for active treatment. Methyldopa was added for those patients who failed to respond to the initial therapy.

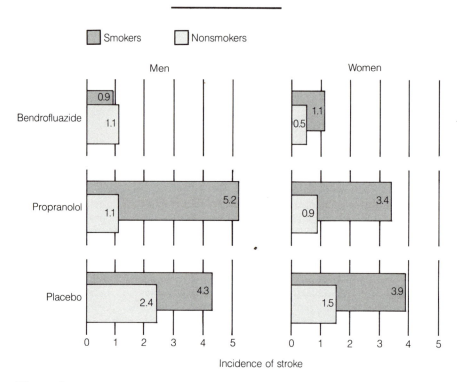

Figure 3.
Incidence of stroke per 1000 person-years of observation according to randomized treatment regimen and cigarette smoking status at entry to trial (from Medical Research Council Working Party, 1985, with permission).

In patients who were treated, there was a significant 27% reduction (p = 0.037) in cardiovascular mortality rate that was due to a reduction in cardiac mortality of 38% (p = 0.036) combined with a nonsignificant (p = 0.16) 32% decrease in cerebrovascular mortality. These data were based on the most stringent intention-to-treat analysis of both the double-blind part of the trial and all subsequent follow-up. When the double-blind segment of the trial was analyzed, a 26% reduction in total mortality was observed that did not achieve statistical significance (p = 0.077). However, active treatment was associated with a significant (p = 0.023) 38% decrease in cardiovascular mortality that was due to a 47% reduction in cardiac deaths and a nonsignificant (p = 0.15) 43% decrease in cerebrovascular mortality. There was a 60% reduction in deaths due to myocardial infarction, and nonterminating cerebrovascular events were reduced by 52%. These are shown graphically in Figure 5. There was no decrement in nonterminating cardiac events.

As pointed out in the accompanying editorial (Editorial, 1985), "One of the penal-

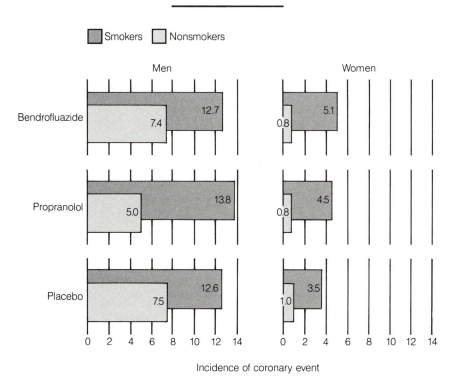

Figure 4.
Incidence of coronary event per 1000 person-years of observation according to randomized treatment regimen and cigarette smoking status at entry to trial (from Medical Research Council Working Party, 1985, with permission).

ties attached to long-term studies of therapeutic outcome is that the treatment initially selected has been preserved as a sort of therapeutic fossil embedded within the trial, so that when the results are analyzed, the drug regimens no longer seem as relevant as they once did." Questions about what might have happened with β-adrenergic blockers, angiotensin-converting enzyme inhibitors, and calcium entry-blocking agents cannot be answered specifically by these data.

Reduction in Stroke The data in the studies already discussed strongly support the concept that treatment of hypertension reduces the incidence of stroke. In addition, an observation on the effect of antihypertensive therapy on reducing the type of stroke was made in an uncontrolled retrospective review of 169 patients hospitalized over two and one-half years for stroke (Black et al, 1984). A group of 44 patients with untreated hypertension had a greater percentage of hemorrhagic stroke than did a group of 47 patients with treated hypertension (52.3% versus 12.8%). In contrast, 61.7% of the treated hypertensives had

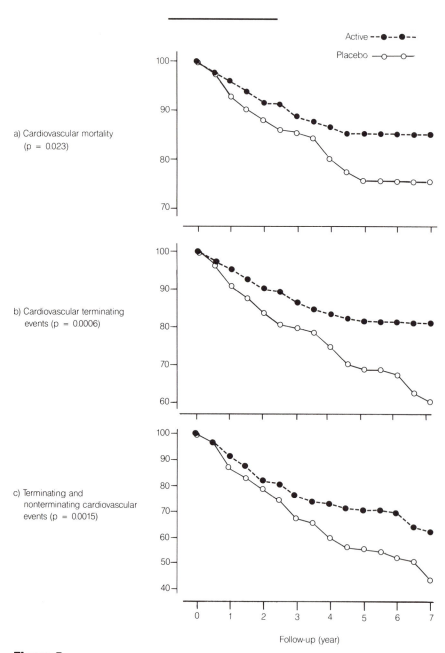

a) Cardiovascular mortality
(p = 0.023)

b) Cardiovascular terminating
events (p = 0.0006)

c) Terminating and
nonterminating cardiovascular
events (p = 0.0015)

Follow-up (year)

Figure 5.
Cumulative percentage of survivors without events calculated for
the patients randomized to treatment by life-table method (from
Amery et al, 1985, with permission).

cerebral infarcts compared with 29.5% of the patients with untreated hypertension. These data suggest that antihypertensive treatment reduces the incidence of hemorrhagic stroke but may be less effective in preventing thrombotic stroke in patients whose cerebral atherosclerosis is already well established.

Cigarette smoking is an important risk factor for stroke independent of age, diastolic blood pressure, and other risk factors (Abbott et al, 1986). Therefore, any study that attempts to analyze the effect of antihypertensive treatment on stroke must also take into account the smoking history of the study population.

Reduction in Renal Disease   There is no question that hypertension is a major cause of endstage renal disease (Sugimoto and Rosansky, 1984). Nephrosclerosis due to hypertension accounts for 18% of the patients with endstage renal disease (Plough et al, 1984). Aggressive intervention with antihypertensive therapy can change the progression to renal failure in malignant hypertension (Woods and Blythe, 1967) and slow progression substantially in patients with hypertension who already have some evidence of renal dysfunction (Mitchell et al, 1980). Most studies of patients with established hypertension and preexisting renal damage show little beneficial effect of therapy. On the other hand, even mildly hypertensive patients have an increased urinary excretion of N-acetyl-β-glucosaminidase, an enzyme derived from proximal tubular cells of the kidney that is a useful marker for renal damage. Successful antihypertensive therapy has been shown to decrease the urinary excretion of this enzyme (Alderman et al, 1983).

LIMITED EFFECTS ON CORONARY HEART DISEASE

Much has been written on the lack of a major impact of antihypertensive therapy on reducing the incidence of coronary heart disease. However, the expectation that there would be a major impact may be unreasonable. Coronary heart disease tends to begin relatively early in life. Factors such as heredity, diet, and smoking play an important role. Autopsies performed on young soldiers killed in battle have revealed a striking incidence of advanced coronary heart disease (Enos et al, 1953; McNamara et al, 1971). It would be unrealistic to expect antihypertensive drug therapy alone to reverse this process. In order to be maximally effective, dietary prevention of cardiovascular disease should begin early in life (Newman et al, 1986). The major epidemiologic studies on treatment of hypertension have generally focused on a middle-aged population whose coronary heart disease was likely to have been well established. Most studies did not exclude patients with known coronary heart disease, and none have focused specifically on prevention of coronary heart disease by blood pressure reduction. The MRFIT group failed to show a significant change by special intervention largely because of risk factor reduction in the control group. It might also have been difficult to single out blood pressure reduction as a single responsible factor had success been achieved.

What is more disturbing is the contrary contention that antihypertensive therapy might, in itself, be a risk factor for coronary heart disease. The two major areas of concern are adverse effects on serum lipids and on the arrhythmogenic potential of potassium depletion. The issue of serum lipid changes remains somewhat controversial (see Chapter II). Nevertheless, it is clear that diuretics and β-blockers do adversely affect atherosclerotic serum lipids and that other antihypertensive drugs either are relatively neutral or exert a beneficial effect. It is also clear that relatively small reductions in serum cholesterol are capable of effecting significant decreases in coronary mortality (Consensus Conference, 1985; Lipid Research Clinics Program, 1984).

The issue of hypokalemia is even less clear. Some authorities provide evidence to suggest that hypokalemia is arrhythmogenic in hypertensive patients and potassium should be maintained at normal levels in patients treated with diuretic drugs or that diuretics should be avoided (Materson, 1986a). In contrast, other authorities argue that studies fail to show an arrhythmogenic effect of diuretic drugs in the face of markedly reduced serum potassium (Freis and Papademetriou, 1986). We (Caralis et al, 1984; Materson, 1985b) have proposed that it is the population of older patients with clinically evident coronary heart disease that is at risk for diuretic-associated arrhythmias in the presence of hypokalemia. For example, the group of patients in the MRFIT study who had cardiac death, presumably associated with arrhythmias, comprised those who had electrocardiographic abnormalities on entry into the study (see Chapter II). Indeed, patients with left ventricular hypertrophy seem to be particularly susceptible to arrhythmias regardless of diuretic therapy (Messerli et al, 1984). In summary, it appears that hypertensive patients without simple clinical evidence (history, physical findings, chest X-ray, or electrocardiogram) of organic heart disease are not susceptible to diuretic-associated dysrrhythmias even in the face of hypokalemia and, therefore, should not be subjected to the risk and cost of potassium supplementation. On the other hand, those patients who are not free from clinically evident organic heart disease should have serum potassium (and, perhaps, magnesium) maintained at normal levels. The reader should be aware that this controversy is still active and that the above conclusions may not stand the test of new data.

DRUG THERAPY CONSIDERATIONS

If the goal of reducing blood pressure is to reduce morbidity and mortality from hypertension-related target organ damage, then the methods utilized to accomplish that goal should not in themselves increase risks for morbidity and mortality.

Nonpharmacologic Therapy   Irrespective of whether drug treatment is eventually needed, all patients should be treated with nonpharmacologic therapy. This includes moderate sodium restriction to approximately 4g to 6g of salt per day (68 mmol to 103 mmol of sodium), maintenance of ideal body weight, adequate dietary intake of potassium (perhaps calcium and magnesium as well), reasonable physical exercise, avoidance of alcohol, minimal dietary intake of saturated fats and cholesterol, avoidance of abuse of any tobacco products, and avoidance of excessive stress (Final Report of the Subcommittee on Nonpharmacological Therapy, 1986). Management of sodium intake and good dietary habits should begin at birth for those individuals who have a high genetic potential for developing hypertension. A no-salt-added diet can be achieved if obviously salty foods, canned foods, fast foods, and most commercially processed foods are avoided. Fresh fruits and vegetables are rich in potassium and dietary fiber and poor in sodium and saturated fat. Unfortunately, this is a regimen that requires considerable discipline to maintain. The same is true of weight reduction. Blood pressure can be reduced rapidly by loss of body weight, and the lowering of blood pressure occurs relatively early in the course of the diet (Maxwell et al, 1984). Weight loss in the first week of supplemented fast was 6.12 ± 0.36 kg in a group of patients eating a 4 mmol/day sodium diet and 4.68 ± 0.58 kg in a group eating 210 mmol/day of sodium. Thereafter, mean weight reduction was about 1.89 kg/week in both groups. There was a marked reduction in blood pressure in both groups in the first week ($-15.0/-9.4$ mm Hg in the low sodium group; $-8.7/-5.4$ mm Hg in the high sodium group). After this initial blood pressure reduction, further blood pressure decline in both groups was asymptotic while the weight loss remained linear. Needless to say, such dietary modifications are difficult to maintain for a lifetime.

The issue on calcium ingestion is complex and controversial (MacGregor, 1985; McCarron, 1985). If calcium supplementation is used, especially for hypertensive women who also are at risk for osteoporosis, then it should be in the form of supplementary tablets or skim milk. Whole milk and cheese products are extraordinarily high in saturated fat and cholesterol. Kaplan and Meese (1986) were extremely critical of the calcium issue and advised that current data do not justify any change in either calcium or sodium intake recommendations.

Physical exercise should be used for general body toning, increasing the feeling of well-being, and helping to maintain a normal body weight (Paffenbarger et al, 1986). Physical conditioning itself can lower the blood pressure on the order of 5 mm Hg to 17 mm Hg (Kaplan, 1983a).

Alcohol intake of three or more drinks has been shown clearly to elevate the blood pressure (Klatsky, 1982). The exact mechanisms are not known, but the excessive sympathetic nervous system discharge that characterizes delirium tremens (and even an ordinary hangover) may be one of the factors. Chronic consumption of ethanol may also induce hepatic enzyme systems that metabolize selected antihypertensive agents, such as propranolol, which could theoretically decrease therapeutic effectiveness (Sotaniemi et al, 1981; Walle et al, 1978). Maximum ethanol intake should be limited to one drink (1.5 oz of liquor or 6 oz of wine or 12 oz of beer) daily.

Many Americans are already well attuned to the idea that consumption of saturated fat and cholesterol is unhealthy. The public does indeed respond to health education. For example, from 1960 to 1983, the per capita consumption of whole milk declined 49.6% to 132.9 lbs while low-fat milk consumption increased from 2.3 lbs to 77.8 lbs. Egg consumption decreased 21.9%, but cheese increased from 8.3 lbs to 20.6 lbs (US Bureau of the Census, 1985). Beef producers are beginning to import European cattle for breeding purposes that are characterized by leaner meat. Considerable attention has been given to the consumption of certain fish oils that contain omega-3 unsaturated fatty acids and that appear to provide some cardiovascular protective benefits from atherosclerosis (Phillipson et al, 1985). Consumption of cod liver oil protects against the development of atherosclerosis in an animal model despite severe hyperlipidemia (Weiner et al, 1986). Reduction of serum lipids clearly has a protective effect on cardiac death (Lipid Research Clinics Program, 1984). Furthermore, restriction of fat intake may minimize or negate the adverse effects that diuretics have on serum cholesterol (Grimm et al, 1981).

Tobacco product use probably has little effect on hypertension per se. However, it is a major coronary risk factor (Deanfield et al, 1984). Carbon monoxide in cigarette smoke might promote atherosclerosis. Cigarette smoking decreases oxygen delivery and may be associated with sudden cardiac death. Smoking may also interfere with the beneficial effects of β-blocking agents (Wood et al, 1978). The MRC trial showed that smoking reduced the benefits of treatment with β-blocking agents (MRC Working Party, 1985).

Stress can cause and aggravate hypertension (White and Baker, 1986). Relief of stress frequently alleviates hypertension or permits it to be controlled more readily. Stress is responsible for the markedly elevated blood pressure seen in patients in hospital emergency rooms and those being evaluated preoperatively. It is exceedingly important for physicians to recognize the role of stress in order to avoid overtreating and mistreating patients. For example, in a study of anti-hypertensive drugs used for the treatment of hypertensive urgency in our emergency room, we found that it was quite common for patients to have their blood pressure fall below our entry criteria during the relatively short period of time that we were engaged in obtaining informed consent, performing the preliminary studies, and obtaining drugs from the research pharmacy. Parenthetically, many of these patients could be controlled simply by restarting them on the drugs on which they had previously enjoyed good control but which they had discontinued abruptly for a variety of reasons.

Preoperative patients are traditionally examined by the anesthesiologist the night before surgery. A certain anxiety level is to be expected and probably reflects normal reality testing. A good night's sleep with the assistance of a hypnotic, if necessary, and reassurance are usually sufficient to bring the blood pressure into a reasonable range. Antihypertensive medication should generally be given in its usual dose on the morning of surgery. Any residual hypertension frequently resolves shortly after the preoperative medication.

Elderly patients with relatively noncompliant major blood vessels tend to show the greatest lability in response to anxiety (Kannel et al, 1980). Small changes in cardiac output or systemic vascular resistance can have a disproportionately high effect on systolic blood pressure in patients with noncompliant vasculature. Realization of these factors can help to prevent unwarranted cancellation of operative procedures.

Pseudohypertension must also be considered in elderly patients who have high blood pressure detected by indirect sphygmomanometry but whose true intra-arterial pressure is much lower or even normal (Oster and Materson, 1986). The clue is blood pressure disproportionately high to objective target organ damage. A positive Osler maneuver (Messerli et al, 1985) demonstrating a palpable radial artery with the brachial artery occluded by a blood pressure cuff is a useful clinical tool in detecting pseudohypertension.

QUALITY OF LIFE FOR THE HYPERTENSIVE PATIENT

As a sophomore medical student in 1959, I learned about the use of ganglionic blocking agents, veratrum alkaloids, reserpine, and hydralazine for treatment of severe hypertension. Serious disabilities, such as orthostatic hypotension, bowel and bladder dysfunction, visual changes, and sexual dysfunction, had made it extremely unlikely that a previously asymptomatic patient would accept such treatment even on the promise of prolongation of his or her life. In fact, about the only hypertension worth treating was that of the severe, accelerated, malignant, or already complicated variety. The patients I saw on the wards as a junior medical student tended to be highly symptomatic and frequently had irreversible target organ disease. Only three years later, mention of veratrum alkaloids or ganglionic blocking agents would evoke quizzical glances from medical students, gales of derisive laughter from the residents, and sharp criticism from the attendings. The advent of diuretic drugs and newer antihypertensive agents had made it possible to treat hypertension without disabling the patient.

Definition and Historical Perspective   "Quality of life is a particularly imprecise criterion subject to misinterpretation and variable application" (Pearlman and Jansen, 1985). "Quality of life" has no inherent specific meaning, and multiple definitions have been offered. Some of these include: "Quality of life may reflect the subjective satisfaction by an individual with his or her own personal life (physical, mental, and social situation)"; " . . . quality of life represents an evaluation by an onlooker of another's life situation"; and " . . . quality of life is the achievement of certain attributes highly valued in our society" (Pearlman and Jansen, 1985). It can also be viewed in the negative wherein one has lost sensory and intellectual activity, personal function, and the essential qualities of being human.

Specific Drug Selection   Specific drug selection may make a difference in the quality of life as perceived by the patient irrespective of the reduction in blood pressure achieved. The patient is unlikely to perceive his or her treatment as being beneficial if it interferes with ability to think, see, control bowel and bladder function, and enjoy a normal sex life (Materson, 1985a, 1986b). Studies performed both in Europe (Hill et al, 1985) and the United States (Croog et al, 1986) demonstrate that the angiotensin-converting enzyme inhibitor captopril is associated with significantly fewer symptoms, including depression and anxiety, and overall well-being when compared with methyldopa or a β-blocker (see Chapter V).

CURRENT STATUS OF HYPERTENSION MANAGEMENT AND FUTURE NEEDS

The Stepped-care Approach   The stepped-care algorithm for treatment of hypertensive patients has been one of the great successes of pharmacologic management of a disease. There is no question that the stepped-care philosophy is effective in lowering blood pressure. One can reasonably expect a 40% to 60% success rate with a diuretic alone, approximately an 80% success rate when a second drug is added, and better than 90% success rate using three drugs (VA Cooperative Study Group, 1977). Most of the major epidemiologic studies have been performed using a predetermined stepped-care strategy for which blood pressure reduction below a goal level (usually 90 mm Hg diastolic) was part of the design. The studies were then able to compare the morbidity, mortality, and adverse effects of groups of patients who were successfully treated with those who were given only placebo or were treated less aggressively.

It is important to recognize, however, that the algorithm itself was a consensus agreement between members of Task Force I of the National High Blood Pressure Education Program of the National Heart, Lung, and Blood Institute. Their report was published in 1973 (Perry, 1973) and was followed by the report of the Joint National Committee on Detection, Evaluation, and Treatment of High Blood Pressure in 1977 (The Joint National Committee, 1977). This group, like the ones who met in subsequent years (The Joint National Committee, 1980, 1984), had representation from such organizations as the American Academy of Family Physicians, American College of Cardiology, American College of Physicians, American Heart Association, Veterans Administration, American Medical Association, National Kidney Foundation, National Medical Association, American Osteopathic Association, and the United States Public Health Service. The consensus was based on as much data as were available at the time and represented a careful and honest effort to make intelligent recommendations for the orderly and logical treatment of hypertension. Keep in mind that the first of the definitive papers showing unequivocable reduction in morbidity and mortality effected by treating hypertension had been published only a few years earlier (VA Cooperative Study Group, 1967, 1970, 1972). Prior to about 1959, medical treatment of hypertension relied upon use of drugs that had a high rate of serious adverse effects. There is another interesting factor. Pharmacologists of that era were reacting to prior practices of illogical combination drug therapy by teaching and generally insisting upon selection of a single specific drug, when available, for a given disease process. Combination treatments were frowned upon. The recommendation of stepped-care therapy essentially presented the message that, under certain circumstances such as the hypertensive patient, combination therapy was not only permissible but preferred.

The Joint National Committee published updated reports in 1980 and in 1984. In each case, they responded to new data that had become available and have revised and expanded their recommendations extensively. Although they continued their support of the stepped-care algorithm, they added a major section on special populations and management problems.

Alternatives to Stepped-care The stepped-care philosophy has not gone without challenge. Some practitioners expressed fear that this was yet another attempt by the government to infringe upon decision-making in medical practice. Others reasoned that equal efficacy could be achieved with fewer adverse effects if very small doses of different drugs were added to one another before toxic effects occurred. This is in contrast to the stepped-care algorithm, where it was generally expected that a maximum dose of each step would be reached before the next step was added.

Another alternative strategy was that of "sequential therapy," wherein one drug would be tried and, if unsuccessful, another substituted until success was achieved.

Therapy may also be selected based on one or more concomitant diseases that the patient might have. For example, a patient with essential tremor and hypertension might be treated for both with a nonselective β-blocking agent (Materson, 1985a).

The advent of the angiotensin-converting enzyme inhibitors and later the calcium entry-blocking agents for treatment of hypertension has focused attention on quality of life issues and has permitted greater flexibility in the strategy of antihypertensive therapy. In addition, the potential lipid-lowering effect of the α_1-selective agents has generated interest in using them as monotherapy. This theme also holds for centrally acting α_2-agonists, such as clonidine and guanabenz, which, in addition to having no detrimental effect on lipids, have a distinctly different adverse effect profile from diuretics and β-blockers. Numerous studies have shown over the years that electrocardiographic and radiologic evidence of left ventricular hypertrophy tends to regress with effective antihypertensive therapy (Samuelsson et al, 1984). The effect may be in part dependent on the drug selected. For example, there appears to be little regression of left ventricular hypertrophy when direct vasodilators, such as hydralazine or minoxidil, are used, but regression has been demonstrated with the use of methyldopa, angiotensin-converting enzyme inhibitors, and calcium entry-blocking agents (Mujais et al, 1983). Angiotensin-converting enzymes and calcium entry-blocking agents have now been shown to be effective as single-drug therapy for hypertension (Massie et al, 1984; Materson, 1984). Finally, a major focus has been brought to bear on the vast majority of hypertensive patients who have mild hypertension and who are least likely to experience early target organ complications of hypertension. It is in this asymptomatic population that drug therapy might very well outweigh the risks of no treatment and where a single drug is most likely to achieve a therapeutic goal.

It appears that the pendulum is swinging again toward selection of a "magic bullet," targeting a selected population subset for a single specific drug. This philosophy has never been tested. To that end, the VA Cooperative Study Group on Antihypertensive Agents is performing a major prospective, randomized, blinded trial on monotherapy of hypertension. Patients will be randomly exposed to either hydrochlorothiazide, clonidine, prazosin, atenolol, captopril, diltiazem, or a placebo. They will be treated for a minimum of one year during which changes in plasma lipids (including HDL subtypes and apolipoproteins) and left ventricular wall thickness will be assessed. It is hoped that this study will provide more definitive guidelines for matching specific drugs to specific patient population subsets and to shed more light on both beneficial and adverse effects of these drugs, all of which are known to lower blood pressure effectively.

Future Needs In a setting where drug therapy is intended to save a small number of people from death and disability due to hypertension by treating large numbers of asymptomatic people, it is clear that the therapy itself must be extremely safe and free from any interference with the quality of life of the patients treated. Medicinal chemists, pharmacologists, medical investigators, and pharmaceutical companies are working toward this end. In many ways, however, the future is now. We have the tools and some of the knowledge at least to approach these ideals currently. Hopefully, new information will help us to use our present drugs more effectively. The information in this book is directed to that point.

Chapter II

CHD Risk Factor Assessment in the Hypertensive Patient: Implications for Management

Norman M. Kaplan, MD

INTRODUCTION

Hypertension is one of the three major risk factors for premature cardiovascular disease in general and for coronary heart disease (CHD) in particular. As a result of heightened recognition of the frequency of hypertension and increased awareness of its role as a risk factor for cardiovascular disease, we have witnessed a tremendous expansion of the number of people identified and treated for elevated blood pressure (Kaplan, 1986b). Unfortunately, as delineated in the previous chapter, the controlled clinical trials of therapy have not demonstrated the expected degree of protection against CHD. Therefore, a reexamination of the association of hypertension and CHD risk, particularly as its therapy may impact upon this risk, seems appropriate.

IDENTIFICATION OF RISK FACTORS AND THEIR IMPORTANCE

Major Risk Factors Long-term surveillance of large groups of people has provided incontrovertible evidence that numerous characteristics and conditions influence the risk for developing CHD (Table I). The best source for such evidence has been the Framingham study (Kannel, 1983). Based upon 18-year follow-up data from Framingham, the major ingredients for the most precise assessment of the risks for CHD have been identified. They are: age, sex, systolic blood pressure, history of cigarette smoking, serum total cholesterol and high-density lipoprotein (HDL) cholesterol, glucose tolerance, and the presence of left ventricular hypertrophy (LVH) by electrocardiography (ECG). Using this information, it is possible to obtain a number indicating the likelihood of a major cardiovascular event developing within the next eight years. Booklets for determining the risk of coronary heart disease and stroke are available from the American Heart Association.

Results obtained with these data, using 40-year-old men as the example, are shown in Figure 1. Notice that as each additional risk factor is added, the

---

Table I.   Risk factors for coronary heart disease.

Immutable	Less strong	Questionable
Age	Diabetes mellitus	Stress
Sex	Heredity (family history)	Serum uric acid
Strong	Obesity	Soft water
(>2:1 increase in risk)	Estrogen lack	**Probably not**
Hypertension	Personality type	Coffee
Cigarette smoking	Physical inactivity	Dietary sugar
Total and LDL cholesterol	Serum triglycerides	Dietary animal protein
HDL cholesterol (inverse)	Ethanol intake (inverse)	
Plasma fibrinogen and	Left ventricular hypertrophy	
Factor VII[a]		

[a] Data limited.

---

probability of a major cardiovascular catastrophe for any given level of blood pressure rises progressively. A 40-year-old "low-risk" man with a systolic blood pressure of 195 mm Hg has a 4.6% chance of having a major cardiovascular event in the next eight years. The chances in a "high-risk" 40-year-old man with the same blood pressure increases to 70.8%.

Another risk score applicable to men has been devised on data derived from the British Regional Heart Study, which examined 7735 men aged 40 to 59 randomly selected from 24 towns throughout Britain and followed for at least five years (Shaper et al, 1986).

The risk score was equal to:

---

5 x age (years),

+3 x years of smoking cigarettes,

+3 x mean blood pressure (mm Hg),

+41 x serum total cholesterol (mmol/1; 1 mmol = 39 mg/dl),

+110 if a diagnosis of ischemic heart disease was recalled,

+110 for electrocardiographic evidence of definite myocardial infarction,

+45 for electrocardiographic evidence of possible myocardial infarction or ischemia,

+75 if chest pain was present on exertion,

+40 if either parent had died of "heart trouble,"

+85 if diabetes was present.

(From Shaper et al, 1986, with permission.)

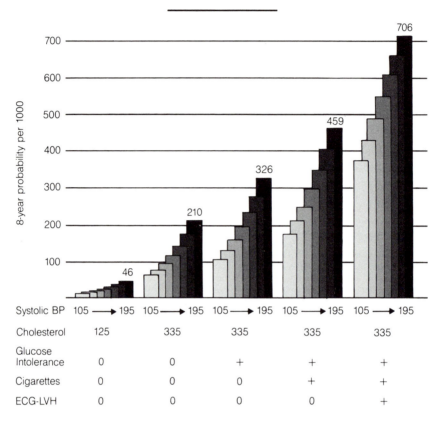

Systolic BP	105 → 195	105 → 195	105 → 195	105 → 195	105 → 195
Cholesterol	125	335	335	335	335
Glucose Intolerance	0	0	+	+	+
Cigarettes	0	0	0	+	+
ECG-LVH	0	0	0	0	+

Figure 1.
The eight-year risk of cardiovascular disease for 40-year-old men in Framingham according to progressively higher systolic blood pressure at specified levels of other risk factors (from Kannel, 1983, with permission).

As shown in Table II, the risk for major ischemic disease events increased progressively with higher risk scores, with 59% of the cases occurring in the top fifth or quintile of the distribution.

Similarly, in the Framingham population, almost 50% of the cases of CHD occurred in those in the upper 20% of risk from elevated serum total cholesterol, blood pressure, and cigarette smoking (Gordon and Kannel, 1982).

Other Risk Factors   As decisive as these data are in establishing the risks for CHD, they must be recognized as incomplete. It is obvious that not all is known. Recall that the independent and important role of HDL cholesterol was identified only recently (Kannel, 1983). Even more recently, a very strong association between CHD and hemostatic function, specifically levels of Factor VII coagulant activity and plasma fibrinogen, has been identified (Meade et al, 1986). According

Table II.   **Risk scores and the rate of ischemic heart disease (adapted from Shaper et al, 1986, with permission).**

Distribution (quintile)	Risk scores (middle of quintile)	Risk rate (per 1000/yr)
1 (low)	775	1.5
2	849	2.7
3	907	4.3
4	961	6.9
5	1060	14.7

Table III.   **Independent associations with all CHD events occurring within five years and over a mean follow-up of ten years in 1511 white men aged 40 to 64 at entry (from Meade et al, 1986, with permission).**

Time period	Age	Serum cholesterol	Systolic BP	Factor VII	Fibrinogen
Within 5 years	1.54[a]	1.17	1.27	1.37	1.57
Over total follow-up period	1.65	1.18	1.32	1.14	1.41

[a] The numbers are for standardized regression effects (SRE), which indicate the increased risk of an event for a one-standard deviation rise in the variable in question. An SRE of 1.50 means that for a standard deviation rise in the variable, the risk of an event increases by 50%.

to the data obtained in this long-term study of 1511 white men aged 40 to 64 at entry, the association of CHD with high levels of these hemostatic functions is even stronger than for increased serum cholesterol or systolic blood pressure (Table III). The association between plasma fibrinogen and CHD was particularly close, and the association of both Factor VII and fibrinogen with CHD were noticeably stronger for CHD events occurring within five years after entry than for events occurring later.

The authors of this study suggest that an appreciable part of the adverse effects of cigarette smoking on the incidence of CHD may be mediated through fibrinogen. Moreover, they call attention to two other prospective studies that demonstrated that the effects of hypertension on both stroke and CHD were limited unless the plasma fibrinogen level was also elevated (Stone and Thorpe, 1985; Wilhelmsen et al, 1984). They go so far as to state that "any benefit on CHD incidence attributable to dietary changes may be due at least as much to short-term effects on coagulability as to longer-term effects on blood cholesterol levels" (Meade et al, 1986).

Whether or not these associations turn out to be as important as Meade and colleagues (1986) suggest, their data indicate that much remains to be learned about the factors that may impact upon the risk for CHD. What is now known can predict only a little more than half of the events that develop over the next five years (Gordon and Kannel, 1982; Heller et al, 1984).

Nonetheless, we need to be aware of those risk factors that have been recognized, in particular those about which something can be done. Even those that are seemingly not amenable to change, such as the sex of the patient (which is arguably the most powerful of all risk factors for CHD), may still be worth attention (Anonymous, 1986). Recall that in the Framingham population, the incidence of CHD in men aged 35 to 44 was more than sixfold greater than in women of the same age (Lerner and Kannel, 1986). The difference between the sexes progressively diminished with increasing age but remained almost twofold at age 65 and 74. The difference could not be wholly explained by differences in the recognized major risk factors. Other data, however, suggest that plasma estradiol levels may be higher in males who have had an acute myocardial infarction, although this may develop as a consequence rather than be a predisposing factor (Anonymous, 1986).

On the other hand, some of the decreasing advantages of women over men with increasing age may reflect estrogen lack after menopause. Postmenopausal estrogen use has been shown to confer a moderate degree of protection from CHD in most, although not all, studies (Henderson et al, 1986).

Interesting relationships continue to be uncovered, including effects of exercise, alcohol, and fish oils. Lesser mortality from CHD has been noted among men who regularly exercised at a level of 2000 or more Kcal per week (Paffenbarger et al, 1986) and in various populations who consume moderate amounts of ethanol at a level of 15 ml to 30 ml per day as contained in one to two drinks (Moore and Pearson, 1986). Preliminary but highly suggestive evidence has shown a protective effect of omega-3-polyunsaturated fatty acids as found in fish oils (Herold and Kinsella, 1986).

Regardless of the role of other risk factors, hypertension, cigarette smoking, and hypercholesterolemia pose the most impact and provide the greatest potential for correction and, thereby, hopefully prevention of premature CHD.

The role of smoking has been rightly emphasized as one element that can most quickly be removed (see Chapter III). Moreover, it stands as perhaps the most commonly encountered risk factor, both for CHD and stroke. Fortunately, the risk falls quickly and markedly upon cessation of smoking (Abbott et al, 1986).

The role of hypertension is unequivocally strong and direct, with a linear increase in risk for every degree of elevation of blood pressure (Figure 2; Castelli, 1984). However, as noted in Chapter I, reduction of blood pressure, as accomplished in a series of controlled clinical trials, has not been accompanied by a reduction in the incidence of CHD. Thus, although the risk from elevated pres-

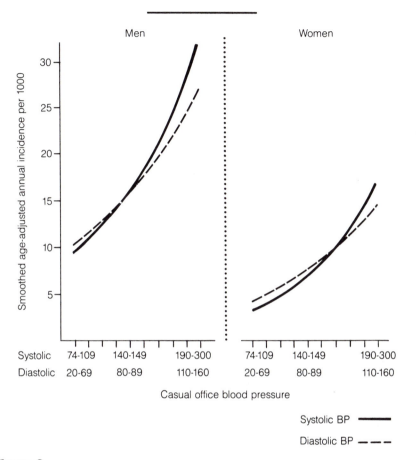

Figure 2.
The incidence of coronary heart disease according to systolic versus diastolic blood pressure in men and women aged 45 to 74 in the Framingham study over a 20-year follow-up (from Castelli, 1984, with permission).

sure is clear, the removal of risk by lowering pressure has not been demonstrated. As noted in Chapter I, this paradox may be at least partially explained by the adverse effect of the drugs used in these trials upon other major risk factors, in particular their effects on lipids, glucose tolerance, and ventricular hypertrophy and ectopy.

These specific issues will be examined in more detail, looking first at the relationship of CHD with lipids, then glucose tolerance, and lastly ventricular hypertrophy and ectopy. With each, their underlying association with CHD will be reviewed, followed by a consideration of the manner by which commonly used antihypertensive therapies may exacerbate and accentuate their danger.

RELATIONSHIPS BETWEEN LIPIDS AND CHD

Once again, Framingham provides perhaps the best evidence for a direct and strong association between CHD and lipid aberrations. These aberrations involve both increases in low-density lipoproteins (LDL) and total cholesterol and decreases in HDL cholesterol (Table IV). Note that the HDL to total cholesterol ratio is the most powerful predictor of CHD, with little added by the addition of other lipid measurements. Hypertriglyceridemia is shown to be a predictor in women but not in men.

Lipid Components and CHD

Total plasma cholesterol The positive correlation between total plasma cholesterol and the incidence of CHD has been amply demonstrated in both within-population and cross-population surveys. Among the 100,032 hyperten-

Table IV. **Relative power of various lipid profiles to predict coronary heart disease in asymptomatic subjects (from Castelli and Anderson, 1986, with permission).**

Lipid profile	Men	Women
Triglyceride	0.51	9.52[a]
Total cholesterol	1.98	2.26
Low-density lipoprotein cholesterol	4.39[b]	4.53[b]
High-density lipoprotein cholesterol	14.03[c]	21.21[c]
High-density lipoprotein cholesterol/ total cholesterol	17.11[c]	20.41[c]

[a] $p < 0.01$.
[b] $p < 0.05$.
[c] $p < 0.001$.

Table V. **Baseline serum cholesterol levels and six-year coronary heart disease mortality in 100,032 hypertensive[a] men without evidence of myocardial infarction at baseline (from Stamler J et al, 1986, with permission).**

Serum cholesterol Quintiles	Range (mg/dl)	Age-adjusted rate/1000	Relative risk
1	<182	4.6	1.00
2	182–202	6.0	1.30
3	203–220	8.8	1.91
4	221–244	9.2	2.00
5	≥245	14.4	3.13

[a]Diastolic blood pressure ≥90 mm Hg.

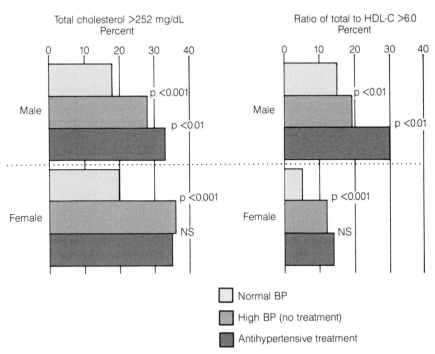

Figure 3.
Prevalence of elevated total cholesterol level and ratio of total cholesterol to HDL-cholesterol in normotensive and hypertensive groups. In all instances, p values or NS designations refer to the significance between one and the next bar (from MacMahon and Macdonald, 1986, with permission).

sive men enrolled in the Multiple Risk Factor Intervention Trial who had no evidence of myocardial infarction on entry, the six-year mortality from CHD rose progressively with increasing levels of serum cholesterol (Table V; Stamler J et al, 1986). These data support a progressive, curvilinear relationship without an apparent threshold. The risk was significantly higher even among those with serum cholesterol levels above 202 mg/dl. In other large surveys, a threshold level has been observed by some (Goldbourt et al, 1985) but not others (Rose and Shipley, 1986).

Not only does total cholesterol pose a risk for hypertensive people, but those with hypertension are more likely to have elevated cholesterol levels and abnormal HDL to total cholesterol ratios. In the Framingham population, blood pressure and serum cholesterol were positively correlated with an r factor of 0.12 (Castelli and Anderson, 1986). Those with higher blood pressure tended to have higher cholesterol levels, so that "half of the women and more than half of the men with treatable hypertension already have an abnormal lipid profile."

Further evidence comes from the screening of a random sample of 5603 men and women in an Australian national study, wherein those with *untreated* hypertension were more likely to have an elevated cholesterol or an abnormal HDL to total cholesterol ratio than were normotensive people (Figure 3; MacMahon and Macdonald, 1986). As will be noted further, the men, but not the women, on antihypertensive drug therapy tended to have even more abnormal lipid profiles.

Low-density lipoproteins   These small particles are rich in cholesterol and are thought to be the most atherogenic species of all the lipoproteins. They are considered to be the etiologic factor of greatest importance in the pathogenesis of arterial lesions of atherosclerosis (Kannel, 1983).

High-density lipoproteins   These particles, the smallest lipid-containing lipoproteins in the plasma, are rich in cholesterol esters and low in triglycerides. Two major fractions have been identified, a larger HDL_2 and a smaller HDL_3. HDL contains two major types of apoproteins (the proteins involved in lipid transport), apo A-I and apo A-II. These have an affinity for cholesterol and may play a major role in removing excess cholesterol from cells.

For whatever reason, higher levels of HDL cholesterol are associated with a lower incidence of CHD (Castelli and Anderson, 1986).

Triglycerides   Most surveys find that plasma triglycerides are less well correlated with rates of CHD than are plasma cholesterol levels. Nonetheless, in the women in the Framingham population, elevated triglyceride levels were significantly associated with CHD (Table IV; Castelli and Anderson, 1986).

Effect of Antihypertensive Therapy upon Lipids
Diuretics   As first noted by Schoenfeld and Goldberger in 1964 and amply confirmed more recently, diuretics tend to raise total and LDL cholesterol. The extensive review by Weidmann et al (1985) clearly demonstrates the effect (Figure 4). Both thiazides and loop diuretics are shown to raise LDL and total cholesterol. This effect occurs rapidly and may persist for at least six years, although some have found the effect to wane after a while. The effect can be blunted by a diet low in saturated fat and cholesterol (Grimm et al, 1981). One diuretic, indapamide, has been found not to adversely alter plasma lipoproteins over a six-to-eight-week interval (Gerber et al, 1985).

The manner by which most diuretics raise total and LDL cholesterol remains unknown, with virtually no evidence having been published as to possible mechanisms. Although it may be in some way connected to hypokalemia and glucose intolerance, one short-term study has shown that cholesterol levels rose similarly in patients given a diuretic, in whom serum potassium levels were kept normal by concomitant use of potassium chloride or potassium-sparing agents as in patients allowed to become hypokalemic (Andersen et al, 1985).

The usual 10 mg/dl to 20 mg/dl rise in total cholesterol induced by diuretics has been shown, on the basis of the Framingham risk data, to counter almost completely the protection against CHD expected from the 10 mm Hg to 15 mm Hg fall in blood pressure that accompanies their use (Ames, 1984).

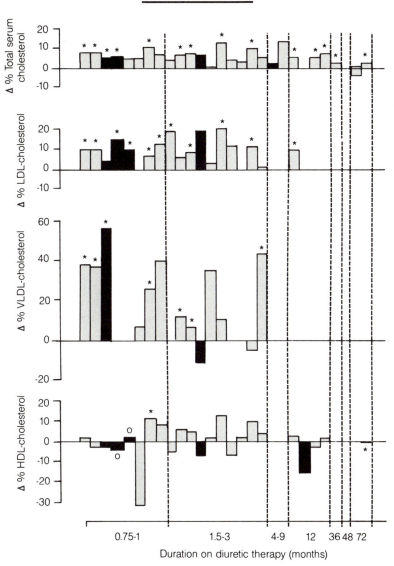

Figure 4.
Percentage changes in serum lipoprotein-cholesterol fractions as related to the duration of monotherapy with thiazide-type (shaded bars) or loop diuretics (solid bars). The data shown are from published studies with a minimum number of ten subjects and a minimum duration of four weeks. Asterisks (*) denote statistically significant changes as compared with pretreatment conditions; p <0.05; and open circles (o) denote measurements by electrophoresis (from Weidmann et al, 1985, with permission).

34

β-Blockers   Weidmann et al (1985) have also summarized the published evidence on the effect of various β-blockers on lipids (Figure 5). With the exception of those β-blockers with significant intrinsic sympathomimetic activity (ISA), namely pindolol and acebutolol, the use of β-blockers to treat hypertension for periods varying from one month to six years has been shown to raise serum triglycerides by an average of about 30% and, simultaneously, to reduce cardioprotective HDL cholesterol levels by about 15%. Although the rise in serum triglyceride may pose little threat, the fall in HDL cholesterol would be expected to increase CHD risk.

As with the lipid-altering effects of diuretics, the effect of β-blockers on lipids seems certain, but the mechanism remains unclear. Some evidence has been published suggesting an interference with lipoprotein lipase activity and a slower clearance of lipids administered to patients receiving non-ISA β-blockers (Day et al, 1982).

α-Blockers   Numerous studies have documented a frequent tendency for total cholesterol and triglyceride levels to fall and for HDL cholesterol levels to rise with α-blockers (Stamler R et al, 1986). Most of these studies involve prazosin, but similar effects have been reported with other α-blockers, such as terazosin and doxazosin, so the effect is probably shared by all agents in this class of antihypertensive drugs.

Again, how this favorable influence of α-blocker therapy upon lipids comes about remains uncertain, although possible mechanisms have been proposed (Sachs and Dzau, 1986).

Central α-agonists   Somewhat less in degree than noted with α-blockers but still favorable changes in lipid profiles have been reported with methyldopa, clonidine, and, most conclusively, with guanabenz (Kaplan, 1984).

Calcium-channel blockers   Limited data suggest that these drugs have little effect upon blood lipid levels (Pasanisi et al, 1986).

Angiotensin-coverting enzyme (ACE) inhibitors   The ACE inhibitors, too, appear to be neutral in their effects on blood lipids (Weinberger, 1986).

To summarize, there are unequivocal associations between high levels of total or LDL cholesterol as well as low levels of HDL cholesterol and the risk for CHD. Hypertensives are more likely to have lipid abnormalities to begin with, and the two major classes of drugs now being used to treat them—diuretics and non-ISA β-blockers—may further worsen their lipid profiles. Fortunately, other drugs are now available that will be either neutral or beneficial on lipids, thereby holding the promise for better protection against CHD when they are used to lower blood pressure.

RELATIONSHIPS BETWEEN GLUCOSE TOLERANCE AND CHD

Glucose Intolerance and CHD   Overt diabetes and, to a lesser but still significant degree, glucose intolerance pose a risk for CHD (Kaplan, 1983b). This risk was shown in the Framingham population based upon elevated fasting or postprandial blood glucose levels. As seen in Figure 1, glucose intolerance is included

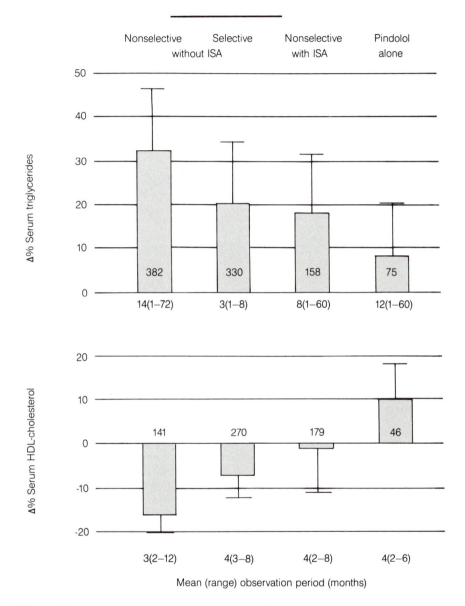

Figure 5.
Mean percentage responses of serum triglycerides and HDL-cholesterol to monotherapy with different types of β-blockers (mean±SD). ISA stands for intrinsic sympathomimetic activity. Numbers in bar columns denote the total numbers of reported cases used for analysis (from Weidmann et al, 1985, with permission).

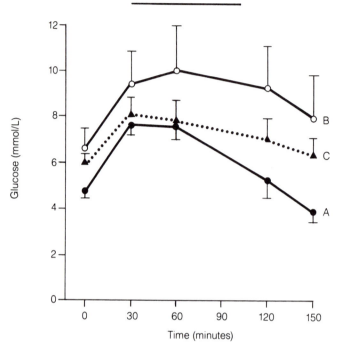

Figure 6.
Results of oral glucose tolerance tests before (A) and after (B) 14 years of thiazide treatment and seven months after withdrawal of therapy; C, n=10 (from Murphy et al, 1982, with permission).

as an independent predictor of CHD risk in the Framingham data base. In a large-scale prospective study of British civil servants, the ten-year mortality rate for CHD was significantly increased in those with two-hour blood sugar levels above the 95th percentile point (100 mg/ml) after a 50g oral glucose load (Fuller et al, 1983).

Effect of Antihypertensive Therapy upon Glucose Tolerance
Diuretics Chronic diuretic usage may worsen glucose tolerance and precipitate overt diabetes in subjects presumably made susceptible by a poor reserve of pancreatic β-cell function. A long-term follow-up of a small group of hypertensives demonstrated progressive worsening of glucose tolerance with four and 14 years of diuretic therapy, with considerable improvement within seven months of its discontinuation (Figure 6; Murphy et al, 1982).

The manner by which diuretic therapy worsens glucose therapy likely involves hypokalemia, either through a direct effect to suppress pancreatic secretion of insulin or through partial antagonism of the effects of insulin (Struthers et al, 1985).

β-Blockers By themselves, β-blockers may cause modest worsening of glucose tolerance (Bengtsson et al, 1984). However, in concert with thiazide diuretics, significant rises in blood sugar have been observed in diabetics given propranolol (Dornhorst et al, 1985).

Of more serious consequence to those taking insulin, β-blockers may block the catecholamine-invoked response to hypoglycemia, thereby masking its recognition and prolonging its duration.

α-Blockers   This class of drugs does not appear to impair glucose tolerance (Shionoiri et al, 1986).

Central α-agonists   Limited data show no significant effects of these agents on glucose tolerance (Struthers et al, 1985).

Calcium-channel blockers   Other than for isolated reports of a worsening of diabetic control with these drugs (Bhatnagar et al, 1984; Pershadsingh and Grant, 1987), most data show little or no effect on blood glucose (Struthers et al, 1985).

ACE inhibitors   Available data show that ACE inhibitors have no significant effects on blood glucose levels either in nondiabetic (Weinberger, 1982) or diabetic hypertensive patients (D'Angelo et al, 1986; Dominguez et al, 1986). In a preliminary report involving eight patients studied by the euglycemia glucose-clamp technique, captopril for ten days was associated with a higher disposal rate of glucose, indicating an enhancement of insulin sensitivity (Ferriere et al, 1985). The authors advise caution to avoid hypoglycemia in patients on insulin.

In summary, glucose tolerance and, even more so, overt diabetes clearly worsen the risk for CHD. As with lipids, both diuretics and β-blockers may worsen glucose tolerance. Although more long-term data are needed, the other major classes of antihypertensive drugs do not appear to affect glucose tolerance in a significant manner in most patients.

ECG AND ECHO ABNORMALITIES AND CHD

The presence of cardiac involvement that may presage the appearance of overt CHD is increasingly being recognized among hypertensives. Until recently, only the rather gross changes demonstrable by electrocardiography were available as evidence for cardiac involvement. With the increasing use of echocardiography and prolonged monitoring of cardiac rhythm, more subtle but nonetheless ominous abnormalities are being recognized much more commonly, even among asymptomatic patients with presumably mild hypertension.

Ventricular Hypertrophy
The risk of CHD   Routine ECG may demonstrate the presence of LVH as well as left atrial abnormalities. Echocardiography, however, provides evidence of LVH much earlier and much more commonly than possible by ECG. In a survey of employed subjects, 145 were found to have borderline hypertension (140/90 mm Hg to 159/94 mm Hg) and 316 uncomplicated sustained hypertension (160/95 mm Hg or higher; Hammond et al, 1986). Using a left ventricular mass index of 110 g/m^2 or greater for women and 134 g/m^2 or greater for men as the cutoff for the detection of LVH, 12% of the borderline and 20% of the sustained hypertensives

had LVH. Although changes on ECG are just as specific for LVH, the echo provides much greater sensitivity.

In Framingham, LVH by ECG clearly was a risk factor for sudden death (Schatzkin et al, 1984) and for myocardial infarction (Kannel and Abbott, 1986). Although slight degrees of ventricular hypertrophy as demonstrable on echo may be considered to be a "normal" accompaniment of elevated systemic blood pressure, its presence too has been found to increase the likelihood of death (Savage et al, 1985) and overall cardiovascular morbidity (Casale et al, 1986).

The effect of antihypertensive therapy   Regression of LVH has been demonstrated with most antihypertensive drugs that suppress the sympathetic nervous system (Panidis et al, 1984), ACE inhibitors (Lombardo et al, 1983), and calcium antagonists (Bouthier et al, 1985). The action of ACE inhibitors may be mediated via inhibition of sympathetic activity because angiotensin II facilitates the release of norepinephrine. Diuretics may do as well as calcium-channel blockers or β-blockers in reducing LVH (Mace et al, 1985).

On the other hand, studies using direct-acting vasodilators such as hydralazine have failed to demonstrate regression of LVH despite adequate control of the hypertension (Bouthier et al, 1985).

The long-term significance of LVH regression induced by antihypertensive agents remains unknown. However, in view of the risk associated with LVH, its regression should be a desirable attribute of antihypertensive therapy.

Ventricular Ectopic Activity (VEA)
The risks of VEA   High grades of VEA increase the risk for sudden cardiac death, which in about 80% of patients is caused by acute ventricular tachyarrhythmia that leads to ventricular fibrillation (Morganroth, 1984). Premature ventricular complexes occurring at a frequency of greater than 10 hr/24 hr or in repetitive forms, either couplets or tachycardia, are associated with increased risk. Some, if not most, of the increased risk with LVH may reflect a greater frequency of VEA noted in patients with LVH (Messerli et al, 1984).

The effects of antihypertensive therapy   Hypokalemia and hypomagnesemia may incite VEA (Hohnloser et al, 1986), and both of these electrolyte aberrations are rather frequently induced by chronic diuretic therapy. The evidence incriminating diuretic-induced hypokalemia as a cause of VEA is increasingly strong but, in some experts' opinions, still not conclusive (Freis, 1986). However, diuretic-induced hypokalemia has been clearly shown to increase the development of antiarrhythmias in patients with mild hypertension and ischemic heart disease (Stewart et al, 1985). Hypomagnesemia may also incite VEA and, if uncorrected, may also preclude the correction of concomitant hypokalemia (Whang, 1986).

The higher rates of sudden death noted in some of the large trials of antihypertensive therapy, as described in Chapter I, may be attributable to their common use of fairly large doses of diuretics without prevention or correction of hypokalemia (or hypomagnesemia) when it occurred. In the one trial wherein hypokalemia was avoided by use of a potassium-sparing agent with the diuretic, the European Working Party on High Blood Pressure in the Elderly, significant reduction of CHD mortality was observed (Amery et al, 1985).

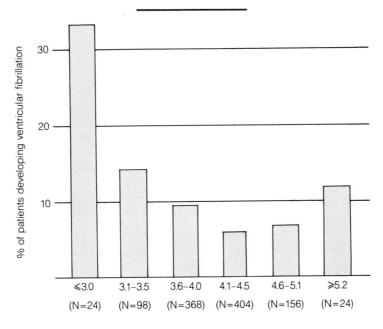

Figure 7.
Number and percentage of patients with acute myocardial infarction developing ventricular fibrillation over the next two days in relation to serum potassium concentration on admission. Of the 117 patients with hypokalemia, 17.2% developed ventricular fibrillation as compared with 7.5% of the 918 normokalemic patients; p <0.01 (from Nordrehaug and von der Lippe, 1983, with permission).

Although the degree of risk from diuretic-induced hypokalemia and hypomagnesemia remains under debate, there is no question that maintenance of normal electrolyte levels is preferable. If diuretics are used, either β-blockers or, even more certainly, ACE inhibitors will reduce the degree of hypokalemia, primarily by blunting diuretic-induced rises in aldosterone, which act to accentuate urinary potassium wastage. If diuretics are not given, neither falls nor rises in potassium, magnesium, or other electrolytes that may incite VEA are expected with these agents.

The special risks following myocardial infarction The greatest danger for the provocation of serious forms and degrees of VEA is after acute myocardial injury (MI; Johansson, 1986). Hypokalemia, whether induced by diuretic therapy or by other means, clearly increases the likelihood of ventricular fibrillation following an acute myocardial infarction (Figure 7; Nordrehaug and von der Lippe, 1983). Part of this heightened likelihood may reflect the further fall in blood potassium levels that accompanies the surge in epinephrine as a reaction to the psychological stress and pain. This β_2-mediated shift of potassium from blood into cells may further depress blood potassium levels by as much as 1 mmol/l. Those who are already hypokalemic might be further endangered by the acute, stress-invoked falls in blood potassium.

Less is known about the hazards of hypomagnesemia in this setting, but transient hypomagnesemia may also occur in the immediate postinfarction period (Rasmussen et al, 1986a). Half of a group of such patients were randomly assigned to receive intravenous magnesium for two days after an acute MI while the other half was treated similarly except that they did not receive the intravenous magnesium (Rasmussen et al, 1986b). Those who received magnesium had a significantly lower incidence of ventricular arrhythmias and of death in the 28 days post-MI. It should be remembered that these subjects were not hypomagnesemic prior to entry into the trial.

IMPLICATIONS OF RISK FACTORS FOR CHD IN RELATION TO THE CHOICE OF ANTIHYPERTENSIVE THERAPY

We have seen that hypercholesterolemia, glucose intolerance, and electrolyte disturbances may increase the risk for CHD and that certain of the more commonly used antihypertensive agents may accentuate that degree of these biochemical abnormalities. Neither the frequency nor the degree of diuretic-induced changes in serum cholesterol, glucose tolerance, and serum electrolytes has been widely appreciated until recently. Similarly, the changes in serum lipids that accompany the use of non-ISA β-blockers have only recently been identified. While there is no proof that the changes induced by diuretics and β-blockers will necessarily lead to the same increase in long-term risks for CHD than would such changes occurring "naturally" from diet and lifestyle, there is no reason to assume that such long-standing biochemical abnormalities, however they come about, will not increase CHD risk.

When we were unaware of these drug-induced abnormalities and when few alternatives for effective antihypertensive therapy were available, there was no reason not to choose diuretics or non-ISA β-blockers, first and foremost. Now, however, when we are aware of these abnormalities and when many alternatives that are equally effective are available, I believe there is good reason to use diuretics and non-ISA β-blockers less and to choose from α-blockers, calcium-channel blockers, and ACE inhibitors as preferable agents to treat the majority of patients with hypertension. Thereby, we should be able to provide all of the protection against CHD that is obtainable from the lowering of blood pressure.

Chapter III

Lifestyle, Hypertension, and the Risk of Coronary Heart Disease: Therapeutic Implications

Robert S. Eliot, MD, FACC,

and Hugo M. Morales-Ballejo, MD, FACC,

INTRODUCTION

The pattern of living for each individual is influenced by various cultural and ethnic norms, economic and social class, personal tastes, and occupational choices. Lifestyle and behavior play a role in many deaths and are a major factor in some of the leading causes of death in the United States. Smoking is a risk factor for heart disease, cancer, and influenza/pneumonia. Alcohol and drug abuse are major causes of automobile and other accidents and are also implicated in cancer, suicide, sudden death, and cirrhosis of the liver. Diet, leading to elevated serum cholesterol or obesity, can adversely affect the risk for heart disease, stroke, diabetes, and arteriosclerosis. Environmental toxins are responsible for certain neoplasms, and such substances may be factors in other life-threatening conditions. Stressors of various kinds can lead to heart disease and stroke as well as to accidents and suicide. Sedentary lifestyle is also believed to add to the risks of heart disease. It is evident that reducing lifestyle risk factors for cardiovascular disease should reduce mortality in general.

Certain aspects of daily lifestyle may be predictive of future health status. For example, Wiley and Camacho (1980) found, in a sample of 3892 white adults under age 70 controlled for initial level of health, that cigarette smoking, alcohol consumption, physical exercise, hours of sleep per night, and weight in relation to height were significantly associated with overall health outcome after nine years.

Similarly, a strong correlation between emotional adjustment and physical health was observed by Vaillant (1979) in a study of 188 men followed for 40 years from adolescence to midlife. Chronic anxiety, depression, and emotional maladjustment predicted early aging, defined by irreversible deterioration of health.

Approximately 40% of the deaths in men aged 45 to 64 are attributed to coronary heart disease (CHD). Because the traditional risk factors of cigarette smoking, high serum cholesterol, and hypertension fail to account for half of the cases of clinical CHD (Gordon and Kannel, 1982), it has become clear that additional lifestyle factors, such as psychosocial stress, coping behavior, physical inactivity, and alcohol consumption play a definite role in its incidence. This chapter will provide information on how lifestyle contributes to hypertension and to CHD. While hypertension is the primary focal point, it is not always easy to separate the data pertaining to hypertension from that of CHD. Therefore, in most cases, cardiovascular risks will be presented in general terms that include both.

CIGARETTE SMOKING

Coronary-prone behavior can be divided into two general categories: behavior related to physical factors, such as activity level and diet, and behavior related to internal factors, such as attitudes, conduct, and heredity. In the first category, cigarette smoking is undoubtedly the most important.

Compared with nonsmokers, cigarette smokers suffer increased mortality, increased morbidity, increased disability, decreased physical function, and increased use of medical care services. Cigarette smoking is the principal preventable cause of chronic disease and death in this country (Taylor et al, 1982).

Hemodynamic Effects   Cigarette smoking causes a transient increase of arterial blood pressure but does not necessarily lead to permanent blood pressure elevation. A study with 19 hypertensive smokers demonstrated an average increase of 11 mm Hg in systolic blood pressure and a 9 mm Hg elevation in diastolic blood pressure accompanied by a 43% increase in pulse rate immediately after smoking two cigarettes (Baer and Radichevich, 1985). These hemodynamic changes were associated with significant elevations of plasma catecholamine, plasma adrenocorticotropic hormone, cortisol, and aldosterone. The increase in plasma aldosterone levels was shown to be independent of the renin-angiotensin system.

Cigarette smoking alone (two cigarettes) or together with coffee (200 mg caffeine) was reported to increase blood pressure for at least two hours in untreated and diuretic-treated hypertensive patients (Freestone and Ramsay, 1982).

In our own study of cardiovascular effects of stress and cigarette smoking (MacDougall et al, 1983), smoking raised blood pressure as acutely as the stress of playing a video game; when smoking accompanied the stressful activity, the effect was more than simply additive.

Most epidemiologic studies report that the blood pressure of cigarette smokers is similar to or even slightly lower than that of nonsmokers. For example, in a study of 2283 persons with mild hypertension followed for five years in Eastern Finland, no evidence that smoking or cessation of smoking had any independent impact on blood pressure was found (Tuomilehto et al, 1986). Similarly, Green et al (1986) found that the lower blood pressure of Israeli smokers could not be explained by factors such as weight, alcohol intake, caffeine, or physical activity.

Hypertension and Cigarette Smoking   Although chronic cigarette smoking is not associated with higher levels of blood pressure or greater frequency of hypertension, deaths due to hypertension are more common among hypertensives who smoke, and smokers have a higher frequency of malignant hypertension (Isles, 1980). It is possible that in some cases smoking may mask underlying hypertension because most casual blood pressure determinations are taken during periods of abstinence; blood pressure has been noted to fall after an overnight abstinence from cigarettes and coffee (Freestone and Ramsay, 1982). In hypertensive patients, a significant association has been found between the past use of cigarettes and the presence of renal artery stenosis (Nicholson et al, 1983).

Hypertensive patients who smoke may be more difficult to treat pharmacologically as smoking can interfere with the effectiveness of antihypertensive agents. In a British study (Medical Research Council Working Party, 1985), treatment of male mild hypertensives who smoked led to a higher rate of coronary events and strokes with propranolol than with placebo. Bendrofluazide treatment reduced the stroke rate for both men and women, smokers and nonsmokers, but caused a slight increase in the incidence of CHD among smokers and had no effect on the rate of CHD among nonsmokers.

While cigarette smokers tend to be thinner than nonsmokers, they significantly increase their risk of myocardial infarction with increased weight more than nonsmokers (Heyden et al, 1971). The obese cigarette smoker triples his or her risk for the development of myocardial infarction in comparison to the slim nonsmoker.

Pathogenetic Factors The increased cardiac morbidity and mortality of smokers may be explained in part by the acute effects of the carbon monoxide and nicotine in cigarette smoke. Although cigarette smoke contains many toxic substances, carbon monoxide may well be the major factor responsible for the increased risk of CHD of cigarette smokers. Carbon monoxide has caused atherogenesis in laboratory animals and binds with hemoglobin 200 times more readily than oxygen (Bass, 1982). Binding with hemoglobin impairs the oxygen-carrying capacity of the blood because during smoking carboxyhemoglobin is temporarily formed in approximately 20% of all circulating erythrocytes. Our studies show that the rate of release of oxygen from whole blood is also markedly reduced. In cigarette smokers, carboxyhemoglobin ranges from 3.8% to 10%, compared with 0.5% to 3.7% in nonsmokers (US Public Health Service, 1979). Platelet adhesiveness and the likelihood of ventricular fibrillation are both increased by the elevated carboxyhemoglobin levels (Bass, 1982). These factors increase the susceptibility to myocardial ischemia, and there is evidence that decreased oxygen release from hemoglobin occurs even in patients with patent coronary arteries (Eliot and Bratt, 1969).

In addition to the effects of carbon monoxide, nicotine contained in cigarette smoke increases heart rate, blood pressure, stroke volume, and arrhythmias, all of which can increase coronary risk (US Public Health Service, 1979).

Since strenuous exercise may precipitate cardiac arrhythmias, especially in a heart whose oxygen supply is compromised by high carbon monoxide levels, strenuous exercise may be a risk for the cigarette smoker rather than a healthful activity (Bass, 1982). Exercise testing shows that cigarette smokers generally cannot maintain maximal exertion as long as nonsmokers (McHenry et al, 1977).

Smoking Cessation Techniques The ever-increasing number of exsmokers in the United States is viewed by most observers as a major contributor to the decline in the CHD death rate over the past 15 years. It has been estimated that more than half of the decline in ischemic heart disease mortality between 1968 and 1976 was related to changes in lifestyle, specifically to reductions in serum cholesterol levels and cigarette smoking (Goldman and Cook, 1984).

Most exsmokers have quit by themselves without professional assistance, although it often has taken several attempts. A physician's strong recommendation to stop smoking can sometimes provide the final push to success. Use of nicotine gum has been found helpful to some people. For those who feel the need of more structured programs, smoking cessation clinics are often helpful. Some are sponsored by hospitals or nonprofit groups at low cost. One advantage of these groups, regardless of the method of behavioral change used, is the support and encouragement offered by others going through the same experience (Terry, 1984).

The major goal of behavioral programs is to produce high initial abstinence rates and to identify strategies that will maintain abstinence. However, as Lichtenstein and Mermelstein (1984) point out, the main thing is to provide patients the skills and the knowledge of how to quit. They advise physicians to emphasize that quitting is under a patient's own control, that quitting is a skill that can be learned, and that, like any other skill, it takes practice, so the patient should keep trying by using the techniques taught in the program. Simple support and encouragement reportedly yield a 15% to 25% success rate at one year (Jarvis et al, 1982). However, nicotine gum used after proper instruction as an adjunct to behavioral therapy can raise the success rate to 47% at one year, especially if participants are encouraged to return for further therapy if they relapse (Jarvis et al, 1982). Nicotine gum also seems to aid those who have been smoking for a longer period of time and have a greater degree of nicotine addiction (deWit and Camic, 1986).

Techniques of self-monitoring, stimulus control, response substitution, and coping skills are most suitable for the behavioral approach. Bass (1982) suggests that the physician write a "behavioral prescription" describing the steps that are to be taken and including the dates the patient has specified for implementing each.

The first step is to identify the advantages or uses of smoking (for example, a way of relaxing, something to do with one's hands, satisfying a craving). Next the patient should keep a record of where and under what conditions each cigarette is smoked; the record could be a paper wrapped around the cigarette pack. As the patient becomes aware of the situations or signals that lead to smoking behavior, he or she then sets goals on which to avoid and what alternate behaviors to substitute. Before stopping, it is important for the smoker to learn to plan for and learn to cope with the situations and stimuli that lead to smoking. For instance, those who smoke for relaxation may be helped by learning relaxation techniques, such as abdominal breathing. Those who use smoking as a stimulant or relief from boredom may substitute some form of exercise, a pocket electronic game, or some other activity for smoking. Stimuli such as a favorite chair or available ashtrays can be removed; stimuli such as the presence of a smoking friend require more difficult coping behaviors.

Indeed, during the cessation period, the patient must adopt a new way of life in order to avoid the places and people associated with smoking behavior. This may mean giving up social gatherings for a time, including office coffee breaks. Then the patient must develop methods of coping with such situations to avoid relapse.

A target date should be set for complete cessation of smoking. Bass (1982) recommends that the quitter reward himself or herself in some small way for each week of abstinence rather than planning a large reward for a distant date.

One impediment to compliance is the fact that most people gain weight on quitting, as smoking tends to increase the basal metabolic rate and to depress weight. In the Framingham study (Gordon et al, 1975), male smokers averaged eight pounds less than nonsmokers, and the leanest were those smoking 11 to 19 cigarettes per day. Men smoking more than this tended to weigh more and to drink more alcoholic beverages. Men who quit smoking gained an average of 5.1 pounds over the next four years. Although differences in caloric intake can explain this, there is substantial evidence to suggest that smoking and nicotine function to lower the efficiency of caloric storage and/or to increase the rate of metabolism, each of which would be expected to lead to lower body weight in smokers. Weight gain after smoking cessation, therefore, could result from the regained efficiency and reduced expenditures of metabolic processes. Also, nonsmokers and exsmokers seem to have a greater preference for sweets than smokers, another factor that may lead to weight gain (Rodin and Wack, 1984). If newly abstinent smokers gain a noticeable amount of weight, they may reduce their food intake and increase aerobic exercise to counteract this problem. Against the background of a newly sluggish metabolism, however, greatly reduced food consumption may be precisely the wrong strategy because too few calories tend to make metabolic processes slow down even further (Rodin and Wack, 1984). An aerobic exercise program that accelerates metabolism may help to prevent or reverse the weight gain.

The final step in the smoking cessation program is to deal with relapse. The goal after relapse is to keep attempting to quit until it succeeds and not to project guilt on the patient during this period. Many good group programs exist. The patient must be reassured that he or she has not "lost" but can return to abstinence, although an occasional cigarette is certainly not advisable. Bass (1982) suggests the use of an "emergency card" with instructions for coping with a very strong urge to smoke: "Smoke this card before smoking a cigarette."

A further advantage of behavorial modification techniques is their adaptability to both public service group programs and self-help programs (Lichtenstein and Mermelstein, 1984).

Community cessation efforts and media campaigns have had good results by creating a climate less accepting of smoking behavior as well as by educating the public on the dangers of smoking and by teaching strategies for withdrawal. Such programs aid prevention, which is the best approach for stopping cigarette smoking.

ALCOHOL

Impact on Hypertension and CHD   Alcohol consumption may account for 7% to 11% of hypertension in men. Most studies indicate both systolic and diastolic blood pressure are elevated in persons consuming more than three or four drinks per day (MacMahon and Norton, 1986). The greater the alcohol consumption, the greater the increase in blood pressure to a plateau at six to eight drinks per day (three to five for blacks). Blood pressure findings in light drinkers vary and, in general, they do not differ from those of nondrinkers. Interestingly, however, light drinkers have lower CHD mortality than nondrinkers.

Abstinence by drinkers has been found to lower blood pressure, particularly systolic pressure, and former drinkers have blood pressures similar to abstainers (Klatsky et al, 1986a,b). Reductions in the incidence of stroke but not the incidence of myocardial infarction are reported to correlate with reduced alcohol consumption. Heavy drinkers who develop cirrhosis of the liver apparently do not develop CHD or cardiac myopathy. Despite the fact that heavy drinkers tend to be smokers as well and to have elevated blood pressure, in some studies, coronary events were less frequent in comparison to more moderate drinkers (Klatsky et al, 1986a).

In general, past drinkers have about the same risk of coronary artery disease as lifelong abstainers (Klatsky et al, 1986a). Heavy drinkers who become abstinent have a lower death rate that those who continue to drink, but if cardiomyopathy is present, not all the effects are reversed (Regan, 1984).

Alcohol Cessation Programs   For patients who are not alcoholics, the aim of behavorial therapy may be to reduce the level of drinking to a moderate level. Alden (1980) described a program for problem drinkers where participants learned a social drinking style that minimized alcoholic intake—sipping drinks, spacing drinks, interspersing nonalcoholic beverages, ordering mixed drinks—as well as ways to refuse social pressure to drink and ways to modify or avoid situations that lead to overdrinking. Participants monitored their total consumption and peak blood alcohol level for each week of the 12-week program and endeavored to increase the number of days that they achieved a self-set level. For one group, the program was enriched with sessions on relaxation and other stress-management techniques. The overall success rate at six-month follow-up was 67% for those who completed the program (57% including dropouts), with a slightly higher success rate for the enriched program.

In treating institutionalized alcoholics, therapy that included training in social skills and assertiveness was found to be more effective than discussion groups in reducing drinking. The behavioral training was done by means of instruction, modeling, behavioral rehearsal, role-playing, and practice in real-life situations. In the year after discharge, the group receiving the behavioral training drank two-thirds as much as the control group and had twice as many sober days, although on the days they drank their intake was double that of the control group (Eriksen et al, 1986).

Because drinking is considered a cultural norm in our society, it would be beneficial for young people, such as high school and college students, to learn the social skills that minimize overdrinking. Education merely emphasizing the dangers of drinking has not notably reduced the amount of drinking or changed youngsters' attitudes.

Certain categories of people should probably remain or become abstinent. These would include persons with an alcohol or drug problem in the past or present, a family history of addiction, and those on medications that can interact with alcohol (Mooney, 1982).

Addiction to alcohol is probably more difficult to counteract than addiction to cigarette smoking. Often exalcoholics will become drug abusers. Sometimes a positive "addiction," such as religious conversion or compulsive jogging, will take the place of the need for alcohol. Such replacements are hard to initiate, however.

To our knowledge, Alcoholics Anonymous has the best record of helping alcoholics to stop and to remain abstinent. However, the individual must first be motivated to change. Understanding what drives an individual to drink can be a clue to the steps needed for behavorial change. The factors influencing adult drinkers tend to be different from those of adolescents. Peer pressure, social pressure, imitation, and mood change are significant factors for adolescents. Boredom, depression, tension, and anger are more apt to lead to drinking in adults (Engstrom, 1984).

Steps similar to those advocated for behavioral change of smoking can be used to change drinking behavior. Stress management, assertiveness training, and relaxation techniques would be valuable for those who drink because of tension or anger. Substitution of nonalcoholic beverages may help those who drink from boredom.

OBESITY

Impact of Hypertension and CHD The Framingham study indicated that obesity is a long-term risk factor for coronary artery disease (Hubert et al, 1983). In this study, coronary mortality and sudden death rates were substantially higher in obese men, and cardiovascular risk increased with greater weights. However, because the weight of Americans has increased between 1960 and 1974, one cannot ascribe any mortality decline to average weight reduction.

Obesity increases the work of the heart and raises the blood pressure, aggravating heart disease in the overweight individual. While early stages of hypertension involve increases in cardiac output, total peripheral resistance increases as the disease progresses. In repsonse to the greater afterload, the left ventricle adapts structurally through a process of concentric hypertrophy. In obesity-related hypertension, the superimposed factor of volume overload also leads to ventricular hypertrophy and adds to left ventricle stroke work. The double overload on cardiac function with its attendant myocardial oxygen demands increases the risk of heart failure (Frohlich et al, 1983).

Three epidemiologic observations link hypertension with obesity: 1) normotensive obese patients have a high risk of developing hypertension; 2) lean hypertensive patients have a tendency to become overweight; and 3) weight loss commonly reduces arterial pressure even when the patient does not restrict his or her salt intake (Messerli, 1983).

PATHOGENESIS: OBESITY AND HYPERTENSION

A variety of mechanisms have been offered to explain the pathogenesis and pathophysiology of hypertension in obesity, including 1) expanded blood volume, 2) elevated cardiac output associated with the volume expansion, 3) associated increase in dietary sodium intake and increased vascular responsiveness to the sodium, and 4) increased adrenergic participation in obesity-related hypertension (Subcommittee on Nonpharmacological Therapy of the 1984 Joint National Committee on Detection, Evaluation, and Treatment of High Blood Pressure, 1986). With regard to sodium intake, a sodium-induced hypertension in Japanese high-salt areas seems not to be influenced by body weight. On the contrary, obesity appears to raise blood pressure via mechanisms that have no relation to the genetic factors of sodium-influenced hypertension (Wessels et al, 1981).

It has been well documented that the relationship between body weight and hypertension is not a fictitious phenomenon of inaccurate blood pressure recording due to an increased girth of the obese arm (Chiang et al, 1969). The use of a large cuff (14 cm x 42 cm) increases the accuracy of indirect blood pressure recording in obese subjects. Although the auscultatory method usually overestimates blood pressure levels in obese persons, there may be a great deal of random variation, particularly in very obese individuals, with possible underestimation as well as overestimation. Tables to correct for arm circumference do not improve the accuracy very much. If consistent values cannot be obtained on very obese individuals by the auscultatory method, it is advisable to use direct intra-arterial measurements before initiating prolonged antihypertensive therapy (Alexander, 1984).

Increases in blood pressure with increasing obesity have been observed at all ages studied. Among college students extensively tested at baseline and followed for 32 years with repeated measures of body fatness, frame, and blood pressure, changes in body weight, relative body weight, body mass index, and measures of skinfold were significantly correlated with changes in both systolic and diastolic blood pressure (Gillum et al, 1982). Nevertheless, baseline systolic blood pressure was the most powerful predictor of future systolic pressure.

In the International Collaborative study on juvenile hypertension, children in the upper 5% of the systolic and diastolic pressure distribution curves (95th percentile and above) were more obese and less active physically, as well as sexually more developed and taller, as compared with the lower group (International Collaborative Group, 1984). At follow-up, the children in the group with the highest initial pressures had a significantly greater prevalence of hypertension and diabetes than the others; also, the incidence of hypertension, stroke, and diabetes was significantly greater in the parents of the upper group. Multivariate regression analysis suggested that weight and heart rate were the main contributors to both systolic and diastolic pressures. Whether the excess weight could be attributed to lifestyle or heredity was not discussed.

A case control study in 121 hypertensive patients and 138 nonhypertensive controls demonstrated that the combination of parental obesity and hypertension is a stronger risk indicator of hypertension in offspring than parental hypertension itself. The authors also found obesity and hypertension in siblings and a positive history of myocardial infarction to be risk indicators of hypertension (Lindholm, 1984).

Weight-reduction Strategies   Short-term studies have demonstrated that significant reductions in blood pressure can be achieved by diet and physical training. In the Chicago coronary prevention evaluation program (Sims, 1981), men with mild hypertension or high-normal diastolic pressure were instructed periodically on risk-factor reduction. Although the average weight loss of 6% of body weight (11 pounds) did not achieve desirable weights, they were able to maintain most of the weight loss for five years and to achieve lower blood pressures. Those with mild hypertension reduced systolic pressure an average of 5.2 mm Hg and diastolic 4.7 mm Hg; those with moderate hypertension reduced systolic an average of 13.3 mm Hg and diastolic 9.7 mm Hg.

Unfortunately, not many people who want to lose weight can maintain the loss for such a long time. It is estimated that 95% of dieters return to their original weight within a year. This is at least partly due to the adaptive mechanisms of the body: the metabolism slows down as intake is decreased, leading to easier storage of fat, and appetite increases when intake is again increased (Leibel and Hirsch, 1985).

Newer studies are beginning to demonstrate that the obese are not a homogeneous group. Some evidently have metabolic disorders, perhaps of genetic origin, that predispose them to weight gain. Specific treatments are being developed for certain subgroups to correct defects in thermogenesis, serotonin synthesis, and other parameters.

One subgroup of special concern consists of those with a high ratio of waist to hip circumference. When fat is mainly confined to the hip and thigh region (female pattern of distribution), it seems to have less adverse consequences than fat in the abdominal region. While fat deposits in the abdomen are more characteristic of males, a high waist/hip circumference ratio is a risk factor for ischemic heart disease, stroke, and death for both men and women. For men, the risk rises for ratios above 1.0; for women, the risk rises for those with ratios above 0.8 (Bjorntorp, 1985).

Although most efforts at weight loss are unsuccessful in the long term, behavioral modification probably produces the most lasting results. Self-monitoring by means of a food diary can be a helpful tool. Entries should specify the frequency and duration of eating episodes and the environmental stimuli that might have led to the overeating. If a diary of eating behaviors shows that snacking or drinking are related to external cues, the individual can devise alternate behaviors with a stepwise plan similar to that described for cessation of smoking. The emphasis, however, should be on success in behavioral changes rather than on weight loss itself. At a clinic using behavioral modification (Sperduto et al, 1986), some groups were told to chart changes in eating behavior while others received the same treatment except for the charting. Members of the former group had fewer dropouts and achieved larger weight losses both at the end of treatment and at three-month follow-up than those in the latter group. Evidently the participants found the feedback of behavioral change more rewarding than feedback on weight loss. This was especially true for those who tended to lose weight more slowly. Also, the system reinforced desirable behavior rather than dangerous behaviors, such as crash diets or use of laxatives, which might have been tried in efforts to meet weight-loss goals.

Behavioral changes can take the form of substituting low-calorie foods for high-calorie ones; confining eating to certain areas, such as the dining area at home and cafeteria at work; refraining from buying rich foods; and increasing activities that are not usually associated with eating. Increasing exercise would be particularly beneficial because this not only takes people away from food, but it can increase the metabolic rate for hours afterward, thus burning more calories and even reducing appetite, in some cases.

ACTIVITY LEVEL

Benefit of Activity   Increased participation in exercise may have contributed to lower mortality trends between 1968 and 1976. Increased activity levels have been associated with lower risk of coronary artery disease in primates (Kramsch et al, 1981) and humans (Fletcher, 1982). Part of this association may be explained by exercise-induced increases in serum high-density lipoprotein levels and by the tendency for exercise to reduce weight, lower blood pressure, and discourage smoking. Of course, it is possible that self-selection may account for some of the correlation between exercise and other healthful habits.

In a study of 16,936 Harvard alumni aged 35 to 74 followed for 12 to 16 years, mortality rates were significantly lower among the physically active. Relative risk of death for individuals was highest for cigarette smokers and men with hypertension, but physical activity reduced the risks even for these (Paffenbarger et al, 1986). The prognosis correlated with the amount of exercise up to the consumption of about 2000 kcal per week.

Recommended Activity Levels   The general recommedations to achieve cardiovascular benefits is a minimum of three sessions per week that include 20 minutes of aerobic exercise at 75% of the maximum heart rate plus 5 to 10 minutes of warmup and cooldown times. Less intensive training for longer periods provides almost equivalent benefit with less chance of injury. Strenuous sports activities have been associated with sudden death. However, a recent conference concluded that even taking into consideration a greater risk during or just after exercise, joggers and other still reduce their overall morbidity and mortality compared with more sedentary persons (Bairey, 1986). Those most at risk for exercise-related death were noted to be men who were not used to strenuous exercise before they indulged in vigorous activity. Among others, there was usually a history of cardiac problems or the presence of an undiagnosed hypertrophic cardiomyopathy, probably of genetic origin.

Most formal exercise programs report good results in increased health and weight loss for participants who stay in the program, but dropout rates are generally very high. For most people, activity levels can be increased more easily in less formal ways, such as by using the stairs instead of the elevator, parking further from one's destination, or taking walks instead of coffee breaks. Many people have found the use of exercise bicycles relatively painless because they can watch television at the same time. We advocate walking as an exercise that can be continued at all ages, can be quite pleasant, especially if friends walk together, and does not require any special equipment. Enclosed malls provide a place for walking in inclement weather.

GENETIC FACTORS IN HYPERTENSION

Evidence for Association Genetic factors are known to contribute to the potential risk for essential hypertension. Adolescents with borderline hypertension and a strong family history of essential hypertension manifested significantly greater increases in systolic and diastolic blood pressures and in heart rate while performing difficult mental arithmetic tests than normotensive adolescents with a negative family history. Furthermore, some normotensive adolescents with only a strong family history of essential hypertension also were hyperresponsive. Hyperresponsivity as well as hypertension thus may be a genetic trait (Falkner et al, 1979).

In the five-year follow-up of a group of 80 adolescents identified as having blood pressure in the borderline range (90th to 95th percentile), 67% had progressed to a stage of sustained essential hypertension (blood pressure greater than 95th percentile). Those progressing to hypertension were characterized by a strong family history of essential hypertension and cardiovascular overreactivity to mental stress (Falkner et al, 1981a).

The association of obesity and hypertension in parents of hypertensive and/or obese children suggests a strong genetic element. The genetic predisposition to hypertension has also been correlated with the presence or absence of a number of varying traits: certain HLA alleles, C3F allele in the complement system, different autoantibodies, herpes virus antibodies, increased adrenal responsiveness to angiotensin II, increased catecholamine release during exercise, and a high proportion of fast-twitch fibers in skeletal muscles (Harvald, 1984). However, screening for such factors is neither feasible nor cost-effective.

About one person in ten is genetically sensitive to sodium, but about half of hypertensives react to sodium. This combination seems to be more prevalent among blacks than among whites (Tobian, 1983), and the evidence of salt sensitivity also increases with age, apparently as a result of defective kidney function (Luft et al, 1983). Even normotensives with a family history of hypertension display increased blood pressure with salt loading and stress (Falkner et al, 1981b).

While environmental factors clearly play an important role in the development of hypertension, twin data and family studies indicate that genetic factors have a greater effect than that of common environment. It is possible that a genetic predisposition to essential hypertension may lie dormant and undetected, needing only the appropriate environmental factors to bring out its expression in adulthood (Williams et al, 1984). Environmental factors that appear to help precipitate hypertension include high sodium intake, low potassium intake, and high alcohol intake. The role of calcium is controversial. While low calcium intake has been reported in hypertensive populations compared with normotensives, this is mainly confined to blacks and is probably related to their greater tendency to milk intolerance. However, in the Kaiser-Permanente study (Klatsky et al, 1986b), total serum calcium showed a positive relationship to systolic blood pressure in all race-sex groups and to diastolic pressure in black men. Calcium supplements have been found to lower the blood pressure for a small subgroup of hypertensives (Lau and Eby, 1985).

Lau and Eby (1985) suggest a hypothetical model for genetic hypertension that incorporates the concepts of various investigators. They theorize that the renal tubule is abnormally sodium retentive before the onset of hypertension, thus expanding the intrathoracic blood volume and eventually increasing the sodium in the cells. Then the circulating inhibitors for Na-K-ATPase would increase, and sodium transport would be reduced. While inhibition of the sodium pump might partially offset the intrinsic renal defect in sodium retention, some vascular tissues would have increased intracellular sodium content. Norepinephrine release would be enhanced while reuptake would be reduced. The increased cellular sodium would also change the transcellular sodium gradient and reduce calcium excretion by the sodium-calcium exchange mechanism. However, there is still a question as to the existence of this exchange mechanism in vascular smooth muscle cells.

MANAGEMENT STRATEGIES

In managing genetic hypertension, it is not possible of course to change a patient's heredity. Therefore, persons suspected of having this tendency should be particularly careful to maintain desirable weight and to have adequate nutrition, particularly with regard to calcium and potassium. Restriction of sodium is not indicated unless the individual can be shown to be salt-sensitive by a blood pressure increase in response to increased salt. For persons already hypertensive, sodium restriction is advisable because antihypertensive medications, such as diuretics and propranolol, are then more effective (Tobian, 1983).

Behavioral therapy for stress management is also indicated because of the spikes of pressure associated with physiological overreactivity in those genetically susceptible to hypertension (Falkner et al, 1979).

PHYSIOLOGIC OVERREACTIVITY

There are many studies indicating a relationship between stress-induced reactivity and hypertension. For instance, rats specifically bred for susceptibility to hypertension (spontaneously hypertensive rats or SHR) react to laboratory stressors with greater rises in blood pressure, heart rate, and plasma catecholamines than do normotensive rats (Folkow, 1982). This hyperresponsivity is detectable even before hypertension is manifest. In humans, studies comparing hypertensive and normotensive patients reveal distinctive cardiovascular responses of hypertensives to environmental stimuli, particularly those behavioral in nature. In addition, exaggerated responses to stress are apparent in young borderline hypertensive individuals (Falkner et al, 1981a) and in normotensive offspring of hypertensive parents (Falkner et al, 1979).

Psychosocial stresses evoke substantial responses of the autonomic and neuroendocrine systems. Some individuals display exaggerated cardiovascular and catecholamine reactions to psychological stressors. Such physiological overreactivity ("hot reacting") has been implicated in the development of CHD and essential hypertension. Psychophysiologic reactivity can be assessed by measuring the changes in physiologic parameters, such as blood pressure and heart rate, when individuals are exposed to behavioral or psychological challenges. Persons who show exaggerated physiologic responses to laboratory stressors exhibit similarly exaggerated reactions to events occurring in day-to-day activities (McKinney et al, 1985).

Role of Stress Stress interacts with other risk factors and can increase their adverse effects. Smoking and stress interact in cardiovascular reactivity, so that the cardiovascular response is greater for someone who smokes under stress than for someone who smokes during relaxation. Smoking may serve to increase the dose of stress to which a person is exposed by decreasing the perception of bodily cues or by improving performance during fatigue or stress, thereby permitting the individual to delay termination of the activity (Epstein and Jennings, 1986).

Emotional stress due to psychosocial conflict and patterns of behavior plays a important role in the pathogenesis of sustained hypertension, renal failure, accelerated atherosclerosis, coronary insufficiency, myocardial infarction, cardiomyopathy, and sudden death (Buell and Eliot, 1980).

There are two distinct neuroendocrine responses to psychosocial stimuli, one being arousal of the pituitary-adrenocortical system, the other involving the sympathethic-adrenomedullary system. In animal studies, social interactions that lead to downward displacement in the social hierarchy may lead to stimulation of the pituitary adrenocortical system with associated mental depression, decreased gonadotropin levels, enhanced vagal activity, gluconeogenesis, and pepsin production—all in an attempt to maintain status and to prevent threatened loss of esteem or objects of attachment (Henry and Ely, 1979; Von Holst, 1972).

When animals are exposed to a life-or-death threat, the animals' reactions appear to be appropriate and teleologically useful. The physiological changes prepare the organism for "fight or flight." Most of the responses appear to be due to stimulation of the sympathetic nervous system and the resultant release of adrenalin-like compounds. Among the most prominent effects are an increase in heart rate, elevation of blood pressure, dilation of the pupils, increased coagulability of the blood, and a shunting of the circulation away from the gut, with increased flow to the brain and to the muscles of the extremities.

These responses would be highly useful to a primitive man or animal exposed to some physical threat. Dilation of the pupils would allow him to see better; increased flow of blood to the brain, arms, and legs would allow him to think better or more efficiently engage in physical combat or provide locomotion away from the scene. Increased heart rate and elevated blood pressure might provide a better flow of blood to areas where it was needed, and it was appropriate that this be obtained at the expense of the gut because it would not be needed at the moment for purposes of digestion. Increased blood coagulability could lessen the risk of blood loss due to hemorrhage.

However, the same reactions used in response to present-day stress no longer are useful and may actually be harmful. Furthermore, factors that cause stress today are much more apt to represent an emotional rather than a physical threat. However, our bodies are apparently still programmed to respond in the same old stereotyped fashion with stimulation of the sympathetic nervous system, release of catecholamines, and other stress hormones, all of which serve no useful purpose in terms of escaping or combating a genuine threat to life and limb. On the contrary, it is obvious that repeated bursts of hypertension, rapid blood clotting, release of fats and sugars into the blood stream, and persistent ischemia of the gut could eventually favor the development of fixed hypertension, atherosclerosis, diabetes, coronary thrombosis, stroke, and peptic ulcer.

For example, repeated physiologic reactions involving excessive heart rate and/or pressor responses to behavioral stressors promote intimal damage through hemodynamic forces, such as turbulence and shear stress. Such endothelial damage is the first step in the development of atherosclerosis (Manuck et al, 1983).

Various studies have shown that catecholamines enhance platelet stickiness and aggregation, further factors in the development of atherosclerotic plaques. Psychosocial and physical stresses have been shown to have similar effects on the platelet (Fleishman et al, 1976; Haft and Arkel, 1976).

Behavioral stressors can exert substantial influences on renal functioning. Shock avoidance has induced significant sodium and fluid retention in dogs, especially in those animals exhibiting the greatest heart rate elevations during avoidance procedures (Grignolo et al, 1982). Sodium retention in this animal model is apparently a result of increased reabsorption of sodium in the renal tubule and reflects sympathetic influences on renal nerve activity.

The autonomic mechanisms may contribute to hypertension through disruption of the regulation of blood volume and the control of blood pressure by the kidneys (Light KC et al, 1983).

In tests with normotensive young adult males, decreases in sodium and fluid excretion similar to those seen in stressed animals were observed as a result of competitive challenges. The effects persisted well after termination of the experimental stressors and occurred only in individuals who showed the greatest heart rate reactivity to the experimental task and had either borderline systolic hypertension or a familiar predisposition to hypertension (Light KC et al, 1983).

Behavioral Characteristics It has been hypothesized (Julius, 1981) that certain well-established behavioral characteristics—hostility, sensitivity, and submissiveness—generate a permanent state of enhanced alertness. This alertness is accompanied by disruption or alteration of cardiovascular autonomic tone, initially an increased sympathetic drive on the heart with elevated cardiac output (borderline and early hypertension). Continued sympathetic stimulation in these individuals leads ultimately to down regulation of adrenergic receptors in the heart and possibly myocardial structural damage, which then results in diminished cardiac responsiveness (normal or decreased cardiac output), and structural changes in resistance vessels altering wall-to-lumen ratios and increasing peripheral resistance (established hypertension; Julius, 1981).

Since Friedman and Rosenman (1959) described and popularized the term "Type A," many studies have been made correlating this behavior pattern with the incidence of coronary disease and with various other risk factors. The behavior pattern characterized by rapid loud speech, impatience, hostility, and competitive drive was originally made using a structured interview. Changes in the way the interview is conducted, substitution of written tests, and problems of reproducibility among interviewers have cast doubts on the relevance and comparability of studies. Also, it is not very discriminatory because more than half of American men are classified Type A in some studies. It has been validated primarily in the demographically restricted group of middle-class and upper-class American men over 39 years of age. In a recent review of the controversies regarding Type A behavior, Dimsdale (1985) suggests that the inconsistency between early studies that found Type A predictive of CHD and later studies showing no relationship might be the result of a change in classification procedures or changes in the populations studied. Since the marked drop in CHD mortality has been largely among middle-class males, blue-collar workers are now the group most at risk. Attempts are being made to determine if certain elements of the Type A pattern, such as anger and hostility, are pertinent in determining risk (Chesney and Rosenman, 1985).

In a prospective study of anger-coping over a 12-year period, Julius et al (1986) found that hypertensives who suppressed anger were, on the average, five times as likely to have died during follow-up as hypertensives who expressed their anger. Systolic hypertension has been correlated with suppressed anger among black males in high-stress urban areas (Harburg et al, 1973) and unemployed white males (Dimsdale et al, 1986).

Stress Management   Awareness is the first step in stress management. Patients must try to identify the situations that cause them acute stress or provoke vigilance. People have their highest blood pressure at such times. A salesman will be most vigilant and have the highest pressure when he is talking to clients on the telephone. A driver watching anxiously lest others try to get ahead of him on the freeway will be experiencing high blood pressure. The simple act of breathing properly during these stressful situations can help lower blood pressure and reduce health risks.

Stress management requires a three-pronged approach: 1) building awareness of the stress triggers; 2) teaching strategies for interrupting the stress cycle; and 3) modifying behavior that accentuates the stress reaction.

Often a physician can identify sources of stress in the course of conversation while taking a careful history. Stressors may occur at work, in the family situation, or from personal assessment. Time pressures, single parenting, and perfectionism are common stressors. In many cases, emotional overreaction is increased by rigid attitudes and irrational self-talks that tend to exaggerate the importance of unpleasant situations. Various daily events may induce self-talks (the conversations we have with ourselves) that are needlessly negative, too perfectionistic, or that lead to inappropriate anger. It is not the events themselves that lead to the emotional and physiological responses but the individual's perception of the event. The perception may be colored by parental admonitions, personal expectations, or mood. Individuals need to become aware of these self-talks and discard those not based on truth or logic. They can then develop more logical, less emotional responses to the same situations. While some events, such as major disasters or the death of a close relative, are worthy of an all-out reaction, most of the things that bother people are rather small. In most circumstances, it is not the events themselves that upset us; we upset ourselves. But individuals can control how upset they want to be and match their reactions to the realities. They can even rate their reactions on a scale of 1 to 10. We tell our patients to try to change a 10 reaction first to a 9 and later to an 8.

Using humor is an aid to lowering emotional overreactivity. Imagining that an adversary is undressed or has a brain tumor that makes him behave badly can have a calming effect. Smiling, even when it is forced, has desirable physiologic consequences and also evokes pleasant reactions from others.

An important part of the therapy is to teach the patient proper breathing by means of biofeedback or relaxation. Abdominal breathing and progressive relaxation are techniques that an individual can easily learn with the aid of written or taped instruction (Eliot and Breo, 1984). For more literal-minded individuals, biofeedback training, which enables them to see actual changes in blood pressure, is more effective. This training requires several weeks of daily practice, however, to be successful.

Time management is another important element in stress reduction. The first step is to determine one's goals and then set priorities. About 15 minutes once or twice a day to evaluate and determine which things really deserve to be done that day can save hours of wasted effort. Another tool is the word "no," which should be used to eliminate time-wasters and activities not relevant to overall goals.

If stressors are associated with particular places, patients can paste colored dots in the areas as reminders to use these techniques. The dots could be placed on the rearview mirror of the car, the office telephone, or even the face of a watch. Of course, rubber bands or other materials could serve as well.

In a program to reduce Type A behavior in postmyocardial infarction patients, Friedman et al (1986) held counseling sessions that included many of the above stress management techniques: cognitive restructuring, recognition of causes of emotional reactions, methods of avoiding or modifying potentially stressful situations, and drills to help establish new habits. The recurrence rate after 4.5 years was significantly lower in the Type A counseled group (12.9%) than in either a control group receiving only cardiac counseling (21.2%) or a comparison group not receiving any special treatment (28.2%).

GENERAL RECOMMENDATIONS FOR MANAGEMENT

Ferguson (1982) sees behavior as a chain of events, starting with a cue or anteced-
ent and leading to consequences that, if desired or pleasant, will be reinforcing.
Antecedents to healthy or unhealthy behaviors can be found in the social environment, physical environment, and cognitive-emotional environment of the
individual. If the social environment dictates a behavior chain leading to frequent consumption of alcoholic beverages or high-calorie food then the social
cues are as detrimental to overall health behavior as toxins or germs in the physical environment are to overall health. Ferguson (1982) points out that the behavioral chain can be interrupted at any point, but the motivation must be
strengthened because the health rewards of behavioral change may be remote in
time as compared to the immediate satisfaction obtained from a cookie or a
cigarette.

Hypertensive patients who realize that behavioral modifications may enable
them to avoid medications have above-average motivation to initiate changes and
to adhere to the program. The physician's role is to teach the patient how to
change, provide feedback about progress, and assist the patient in planning and
reinforcing health-enhancing behaviors. When individuals become involved in
their own health care and realize that they have the primary responsibility for
the outcome, they tend to implement behavioral changes on their own.

As may already be apparent, behavior modification—whatever the goal—consists
of the same basic steps. First, identification of the cues or situations leading to
the undesirable behavior; second, planning on how to modify or replace the undesirable behavior, including a timetable for instituting the changes; third, feedback on improvement through self-monitoring and encouragement from
physician, counselor, and/or family; and fourth, relapse prevention.

The individual must be able to envision the needed changes as a series of achiev-
able goals. He or she must also be fortified with rehearsed techniques for dealing
with temptation and with relapses. If several behaviors, such as cigarette smoking and emotional overreacting, need to be altered, the first change should be the
one easiest for the patient to achieve. When this change has been made, a pattern
of successful accomplishment will have been established. Expectation of success
breeds success.

Patient involvement and compliance can be increased by having him or her sign
a written contract stating what is to be accomplished. This is a way of enhancing
motivation and arranging for systematic reinforcement of behaviors contingent
upon performance. This type of contract can be between the physician and the
patient, the patient and his family, or the patient and himself (perhaps with a set
reward).

Self-monitoring to provide feedback can take various forms: graphs, charts, di-
aries, or marks on a diagram or calendar. Ferguson (1982) finds that "the more
novel the feedback system, the more interested the patient will be, and the more
the feedback demonstrates progress and enhances self-efficacy, the better the
therapeutic effect." In all cases, it is necessary to explain the goals and reasons
for treatment to the patient, who must agree with the physician that the pro-

posed goals are appropriate and desirable. It takes time for new behaviors to become habitual. Follow-up periodically for at least six months may be necessary to assure long-term compliance.

Relaxation breaks, optimal activity level, and positive self-talks are helpful to everyone, regardless of their behavioral problems. Social support is a necessity for most people. Joining a group of others with the same problem can provide social support and aid compliance. Organizations for those trying to deal with addictions, overweight, or family problems can be located through a hospital social service department or even the telephone directory.

CONCLUSIONS

Hypertension is one of the most prevalent and costly diseases in the western world. The use of behavioral means to control and to prevent high blood pressure offers potential benefits on cost of therapy and quality of life in patients who respond. Delay in prescribing medications may therefore be wise in the case of mild hypertension because normalization may occur spontaneously. Behavioral modification can also be of benefit in patients whose blood pressure is not completely controlled by this means because it can reduce medication requirements. In addition, an improved lifestyle instituted for a hypertensive patient may improve the health of the whole family, preventing or delaying development of cardiovascular illness in the younger generation.

ACKNOWLEDGMENTS

The editorial effort for this chapter was supported by the International Stress Foundation and the Monsour Medical Foundation.

Chapter IV

Hemodynamics in the Patient with Hypertension at Rest and During Exercise: Impact of Antihypertensive Therapy

Michael A. Weber, MD, and William F. Graettinger, MD

INTRODUCTION

It is difficult to be specific in defining mechanisms responsible for sustaining hypertension for there are many factors that can work directly or through interactions with other factors to influence blood pressure. Neuronal and hormonal systems originating from the central nervous system, heart, kidneys, adrenal cortex, and medulla and from vascular tissue itself can participate in differing ways in the genesis of high blood pressure. Clinically, it has been possible to draw some broad generalizations. Because various types of antihypertensive therapy appear to have their optimal effects in differing demographic subgroups, it has been suggested that mechanisms sustaining hypertension in older patients may be different from those in the young, and mechanisms of hypertension in black patients may be different from those in whites. It has also been shown that mechanisms of hypertension might change within individuals as they grow older. Moreover, the use of antihypertensive pharmacology often evokes compensatory hemodynamic mechanisms that can alter the initial hemodynamic profile.

For these reasons, it is probably most appropriate to look at hemodynamic factors at rest and during exercise in hypertensive patients on an empirical basis rather than trying to fully define the underlying regulatory mechanisms that govern these parameters. In this chapter, the hemodynamic characteristics of the untreated hypertensive patient at rest and during exercise will be examined. The effects of the differing classes of antihypertensive agents on exercise performance will then be discussed. Consideration will be given not only to the younger, generally healthy individual who wishes to undertake a fairly rigorous conditioning program but also to the hypertensive patient whose activity is limited by ischemic heart disease.

Hemodynamic Patterns in Early and Late Hypertension A fundamental tenet of hemodynamics is that blood pressure is equal to the product of cardiac output and total peripheral resistance. Both blood pressure and cardiac output can be measured directly by invasive or noninvasive methods, thereby allowing the total peripheral resistance to be calculated algebraically. There is no practical method in either clinical or whole-animal investigation to directly measure peripheral resistance for it is thought to reflect largely the state of constriction of the small arterioles and precapillary sphincters that comprise the terminal arterial circulation. Based on this simple model of hemodynamics, hypertension can result from an increase in cardiac output, an increase in peripheral resistance, or possibly both.

There is evidence to suggest that hypertension in younger patients, typically less than 40 years old, may be associated primarily with increases in cardiac output. Table I summarizes data from four studies in which values for mean arterial blood pressure, cardiac index, and total peripheral resistance were obtained in younger patients with mild essential hypertension. In each of these studies (Bello et al, 1965; Frohlich et al, 1969; Lund-Johansen, 1967; Weiss et al, 1973), cardiac index was higher in hypertensive individuals than in age-matched normotensive controls. Although cardiac output is the product of heart rate and stroke volume, findings in these studies indicated that increased cardiac index values were due to increases in heart rate alone because stroke index was similar in hypertensive and normotensive individuals. In a further study in young patients with very early evidence of hypertension, total peripheral resistance was actually slightly reduced, and their hypertension was due entirely to a marked increase in cardiac output (Safar et al, 1973). This type of mild hypertension in the young, characterized clinically by a relative tachycardia, is sometimes termed hyperadrenergic hypertension. The pattern of increased chronotropic drive to the heart, associated with normal arterial tone or perhaps even a slight dilation, is somewhat suggestive of increased epinephrine-like activity. Not surprisingly, the β-adrenergic blocking agents, which pharmacologically are comparatively specific antagonists of epinephrine, have been found to be highly effective therapeutically in this type of early hypertension.

Hypertension in middle-aged and older patients generally has a different hemodynamic profile; cardiac output is normal or even slightly decreased (Lund-Johansen, 1967; Safar et al, 1973), and hypertension is due to increased peripheral resistance. As hypertension becomes more severe at any age, there is a tendency for cardiac output to fall further, chiefly as a result of a reduction in stroke volume. Under these circumstances, there may even be a slight increase in heart rate, but it is insufficient to compensate for the reduced stroke volume. Obviously, the hypertension in these patients is characterized by marked increases in total peripheral resistance (Frohlich et al, 1969; Lund-Johansen, 1967).

Most studies of hemodynamics in hypertension inevitably have been cross-sectional in nature, studying untreated patients at a single instance in time. However, longitudinal observations in hypertensive cohorts have provided some interesting information (Lund-Johansen, 1978b; Weiss et al, 1973). In one such study, 28 young patients (18 to 39 years old at the start of the observation) were followed for ten years (Lund-Johansen, 1978b). At the end of this period, blood

Table I. **Average hemodynamic values in young, mildly hypertensive patients (H) and normotensive controls (C) reported from four separate studies (from Lund-Johansen, 1980, with permission).**

Reference	Mean arterial pressure (mm Hg)		Cardiac index (1/min/m^2)		Heart rate (bpm)		Stroke index (ml/beat m^2)		Total peripheral resistance index (K Pa sec 1^{-1}m^2)	
	H	C	H	C	H	C	H	C	H	C
Bello et al, 1965	108	91	4.1	3.3	81	74	51	44	211	221
Frohlich et al, 1969	106	93	3.5	3.1	77	68	46	45	240	244
Lund-Johansen, 1967	102	84	4.1	3.5	75	63	56	55	197	195
Weiss et al, 1973	100	87	4.2	3.7	77	72	55	52	201	194

pressure had not changed significantly, but average cardiac output was lower than at the start of the study and total peripheral resistance had increased. Thus, differences between younger and older hypertensive hemodynamic patterns observed in the cross-sectional studies were paralleled by the transition in hemodynamic parameters within the untreated mild hypertensive studied longitudinally. Another interesting conclusion was reached in this study based on the further observation that the differing early and later hemodynamic profiles observed within the patients followed for ten years were not reflected by differences obtained in separate observations of two other groups of hypertensives with a ten-year age difference between them (Lund-Johansen, 1978b). This finding suggested that age alone may not be the basis for the differing hemodynamic patterns in older and younger patients but rather that the progressive rise in peripheral resistance (and the secondary fall in the cardiac output) might be due partly to effects of hypertension itself on vascular tissue.

The Heart and Kidneys It is possible that the changing hemodynamic picture seen as the hypertensive patient ages might have an impact on the heart itself. There is evidence that older patients are more likely than younger patients to have large hearts, especially left ventricular hypertrophy (Kannel et al, 1969). It could be argued that the growing importance of peripheral resistance, or cardiac afterload, with the progression of hypertension places a continuously greater contractile demand on the myocardium. Thus, a modest degree of left ventricular muscle hypertrophy could be regarded as an adaptive change required to ensure the maintenance of cardiac output and the adequate perfusion of vital organs.

It is important to note that high blood pressure is not the only stimulus to cardiac hypertrophy. Other key factors contributing to development of hypertrophy are increased sympathetic drive, activity of the renin-angiotensin system, and increased viscosity of blood (Weber et al, 1986). The tendency for older hypertensive patients to have left ventricular hypertrophy is consistent with the observation that these individuals appear to have heightened vascular responsiveness to activity of the sympathetic nervous system (Palmer et al, 1978). Moreover, *in vivo* and *in vitro* studies with myocardial tissue have also shown the importance of adrenergic stimuli in activating hypertrophic changes (Weber et al, 1986). The differential effects of antihypertensive drugs on cardiac size have supported this hypothesis. Agents that block sympathetic drive, such as methyldopa or clonidine, have been shown to cause regression of left ventricular hypertrophy even when they fail to decrease blood pressure (Arevalo, 1983; Drayer et al, 1982a). Similarly, the converting-enzyme inhibitors, which block the renin-angiotensin system and may additionally have some antisympathetic action as well, have been shown to cause regression of hypertrophy in hypertensive patients (McKenna et al, 1982; Ventura et al, 1985). On the other hand, agents such as diuretics or direct-acting vasodilators, which often are effective antihypertensive drugs but which may actually stimulate sympathetic or renin factors, generally fail to reverse hypertrophic changes (Drayer et al, 1982b; Frohlich and Tarazi, 1979).

Renal function as measured by glomerular filtration rate usually is normal in hypertensive patients except in those with severe forms of the disease. Renal blood flow, however, has an interesting pattern that parallels the changes in cardiac output with increasing age. In young patients, especially those aged less than 30 years, renal blood flow, like cardiac output, might actually be greater than in age-matched normotensive controls, but at later ages the renal blood flow falls to within the normal range (Messerli et al, 1981b; Temmar et al, 1981). In patients with more severe forms of hypertension, and particularly in older patients, there may be a tendency for renal blood flow to fall below normal levels (Temmar et al, 1981). Renal blood flow is the result of many complex intrarenal vascular regulatory systems. Although blood flow to the kidney in young patients appears to reflect the hemodynamics of the systemic circulation, it is likely that intrarenal hormonal, neuronal, and mechanical factors later become the dominant determinants of renal blood flow.

Further participation factors in hemodynamics are fluid volume and sodium. As with the changes in patterns of cardiac output and total peripheral resistance, the volume picture also seems to change with age. Younger patients, when compared with normotensive age-matched controls, may actually be slightly volume and sodium depleted (Beretta-Piccoli et al, 1982). Presumably, these measurements, obtained by radionuclide methods, reflect the physiologically appropriate pressure natriuresis exerted by the kidneys in response to the elevation in blood pressure. In older patients, plasma volume and total body sodium measurements return to normal or sometimes may even be in a slightly expanded state.

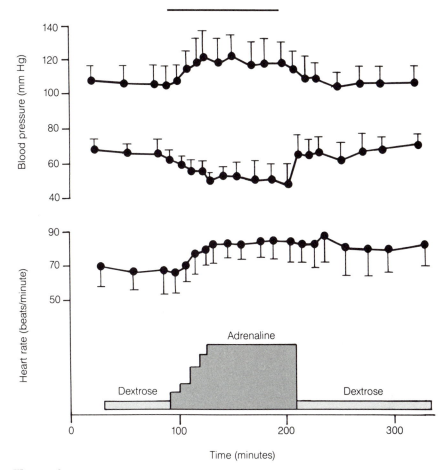

Figure 1.
Effects on blood pressure and heart rate of epinephrine (adrenaline)
infused at a maximum rate of 0.06 mg/kg/min in eight normal
volunteers. Values are mean ± SD (from Reid et al, 1986, with
permission).

EFFECTS OF EXERCISE

Exercise is a form of physical stress that requires hemodynamic and metabolic adaptations. In the healthy individual, major changes normally occur only with fairly severe grades of exercise, but even mild exertion can require substantial changes in patients with underlying cardiac disease. Hypertension also can influence hemodynamic adaptations to exercise.

In the healthy young individual, the initial hemodynamic response to dynamic exercise is characterized by modest increases in systolic blood pressure and heart rate and by a small reduction or no change in diastolic blood pressure (Wolthins et al, 1977). It is likely that systematic physical training programs can modify the pressor response to exercise (Sannerstedt et al, 1973). In some respects, this profile is identical to that associated with the physiologic or pharmacologic effects of epinephrine, as shown in Figure 1 (Reid et al, 1986). These data, obtained in young volunteers, show the effects of epinephrine infused in amounts similar to those likely to be stimulated during conditions of stress or exercise. In man, this effect is likely to be mediated through activation primarily of β_2-receptors, which have both chronotropic and inotropic effects on the heart but which also mediate vasodilation of the peripheral arterial circulation (Stene-Larsen et al, 1986). These receptors also mediate the epinephrine-induced rapid cellular uptake of potassium observed during physical stress, possibly leading to hypokalemia; potentially, this could lead to clinically adverse events such as dysrhythmias in patients with underlying ischemic heart disease. Clearly, in patients with hypertension or other forms of cardiovascular disease, it is desirable that exercise not be associated with excessive increases in blood pressure, heart rate, or catecholamines and the metabolic changes such as those with potassium be kept to a minimum.

Blood pressure responses to graded exercise in patients with essential hypertension are shown in Figure 2 (Taylor, 1980). These increases are probably greater than those observed in normotensive individuals. It has also been suggested that patients with apparently normal blood pressures, but whose systolic levels exceed 225 mm Hg during treadmill exercise, have a greater likelihood of subsequently becoming hypertensive than those whose blood pressures increase less markedly (Wilson and Meyer, 1981). Increases in diastolic pressures during exercise also may have prognostic significance.

Isometric exercise, such as handgrip testing or lifting or straining, increases both systolic and diastolic blood pressures in normal individuals, probably mediated by a marked reduction in vagal tone (Riendl et al, 1977). This response may be exaggerated in hypertensive patients (Ewing et al, 1973). As discussed later, there are few if any forms of antihypertensive therapy that can protect against these sharp rises in blood pressure, and it is thus considered prudent to advise hypertensive patients to minimize this type of exertion.

A fundamental need with exercise is the delivery of adequate amounts of oxygen and energy-providing substances to the exercising muscles. This demands hemodynamic changes that increase cardiac output and cause vasodilation. Although there may be some increase in systolic blood pressure, the predominant hemodynamic change should be an increase in cardiac output, preferably associated with a modest reduction in peripheral resistance (Lund-Johansen, 1980). A goal of antihypertensive treatment, apart from decreasing blood pressure at rest, is to preserve the appropriate hemodynamic profile at times of exercise. It is likely, however, that differences in the effects of drugs, which perhaps are only minimal at rest, become more evident during exercise. For example, treatment with agents such as α_1-blockers and β-blockers can produce distinctly different hemodynamic effects. The α-blockers decrease total peripheral resistance but do not alter cardiac output at rest; with exercise, however, there is an appropriate increase in cardiac output, and peripheral resistance may decrease even further (Lund-Johansen, 1975). In contrast,

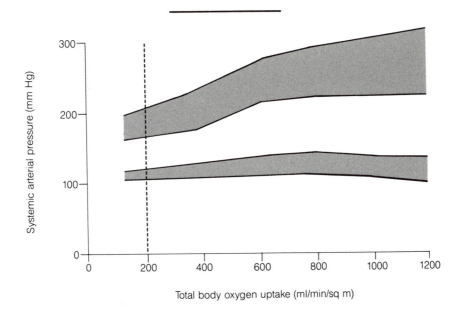

Figure 2.
Effects on systolic and diastolic blood pressures of increasing levels of treadmill exercise in patients with essential hypertension. The shaded areas indicate the mean ±2 SD of the blood pressure responses (from Taylor, 1980, with permission).

β-blockers usually decrease cardiac output at rest and, importantly, may limit the increase normally stimulated by exercise (Lund-Johansen, 1976).

It is important to note that questions of exercise and physical work may be completely different in patients with underlying ischemic heart disease. In such patients, it may be desirable to put limitations on cardiac work, which approximates the product of heart rate and systolic blood pressure. In the presence of coronary artery disease, ability of drugs such as β-blockers to decrease oxygen demand by the myocardium might actually enable moderate degrees of exercise to be carried out. Thus, despite their apparently negative impact on exercise challenges in otherwise healthy hypertensive patients, β-blockers may be of considerable value in hypertensive patients who concurrently have underlying coronary disease.

Metabolic Aspects of Exercise   Physical exercise evokes a number of metabolic changes in order to provide energy to the heart and the exercising skeletal muscles. Cardiac work increases considerably during exercise because of the increases in both heart rate and stroke volume. Early in the course of dynamic exercise, the myocardium responds by increasing its uptake of glucose and lactate; it is likely that lactate is the preferred energy source for the myocardium during the earlier phase of exercise. But as dynamic activity is prolonged, there is a tendency for lactate supply to diminish owing possibly to a reduced availability from muscle glycogen sources. Competitive athletes, exemplified by marathon runners, sometimes try dietary strategies such as "glycogen loading" in an attempt to prolong this form of energy during their exercise. Once this source has been depleted, however, free fatty acids become the main energy available to the myocardium. Additionally, endogenous lipolysis produces glycerol, which also contributes to the energy pool available to the myocardium (Kaijser et al, 1972).

Skeletal muscle has major metabolic demands of its own during exercise. Local blood flow to the exercising muscle usually increases quite markedly, but despite the availability of free fatty acids and glucose from this increasing circulatory supply, local glycogen breakdown in the muscle becomes an increasingly important source of energy during more protracted exercise. To an important extent, the availability of glucose to the myocardium and skeletal muscle is dependent upon effective hepatic glycogenolysis. Except in patients with dietary deficiencies or in the presence of liver disease, this source of energy is not usually a limiting factor in exercise.

During prolonged exercise, free fatty acids become an important source of energy for both the myocardium and skeletal muscle. They originate from the breakdown of triglycerides, which is largely an adrenergic function. This mechanism becomes of considerable importance to athletes or other individuals who undertake serious training programs, for it is likely that one of the effects of training is stimulation of skeletal muscle mitochondria, which results in an enhanced ability of muscle tissue to utilize free fatty acids as a source of energy. It is possible, too, that regular use of adipose tissue as an energy source during regular training or conditioning might confer additional benefits. Because of the importance of oxygen in most of these energy-generating metabolic processes, a key part of the overall metabolic and hemodynamic response to exercise is an increase in ventilatory function.

These metabolic and hemodynamic responses are the key to successfully undertaking short-term or long-term programs of physical activity. Although various mechanisns may participate in mediating these changes, the peripheral sympathetic or adrenergic system clearly has a pivotal role. This has practical significance during antihypertensive therapy. The various classes of agents have differing effects on adrenergic and other mechanisms that participate in the response and may thereby alter the physical performance of the treated patient.

ANTIHYPERTENSIVE AGENTS

There are two ways of regarding the effects of antihypertensive drugs on hemodynamics. The first is to evaluate their actions in hypertensive patients at rest, and the second is to determine the ways in which they might modify, if at all, the normal hemodynamic responses to exercise. Although most investigators have studied dynamic rather than static exercise, it is of some interest and practical value to consider the effects of treatment on blood pressure responses to isometric stimuli, such as sustained handgrip or lifting. Because there are marked differences between the drug classes in their effects (Lowenthal and Kendrick, 1985), it is most useful to consider them separately.

Diuretic Agents The diuretic agents have been used as first-line therapy for the treatment of hypertension for several years. They are effective both as single-agent therapy and as part of combination treatment with other antihypertensive drugs. The emergence of other agents that are at least as effective as diuretics in decreasing blood pressure, together with concerns over possible deleterious effects of the metabolic actions of diuretics, has led to some reduction in their use. However, their relative freedom from causing severe symptomatic side effects, the convenience of once-daily dosing in most patients, and their inexpensiveness has continued to maintain interest in using these agents as first-line treatment.

The initial effect of diuretics is to produce natriuresis, which results in volume depletion as measured by decreases in blood and plasma volume. In turn, there is a reduction in cardiac output and renal perfusion. Total peripheral resistance remains the same or may actually increase during this early phase of treatment (Diakonova and Iurenev, 1982; Roos et al, 1981). However, after several weeks or months of treatment, there is a tendency for the cardiac output to increase to its pretreatment control levels and for total peripheral resistance to fall (Lund-Johansen, 1970). Thus, during long-term therapy with diuretics, the hemodynamic picture, at least in the resting patient, appears to be desirable because the principal hemodynamic abnormality of hypertension, namely the increased peripheral resistance, is reduced. However, the fundamental pharmacologic action of the diuretics is through their ability to produce sodium and water depletion, and measurements of fluid volume verify this reduction (Shah et al, 1978). Moreover, even after a year of treatment with diuretics, there is still a tendency in some patients to have a cardiac index that has not quite returned to a normal level and for the peripheral resistance to be only slightly decreased (Lund-Johansen, 1970).

It is likely that the transition from the early decrease in cardiac output toward the later normalization is mediated through various autoregulatory mechanisms. These apparently corrective trends may be opposed by the effects of the continuing volume depletion on the renin-angiotensin-aldosterone system and the sympathetic nervous system. The reactive changes in these two systems ultimately increase levels of angiotensin II and norepinephrine, both of which mediate vasoconstrictor effects. These effects, in turn, are likely to sustain increased total peripheral resistance and thereby retard the reversion of the hemodynamic profile to normal. The compensatory neuroendocrine mechanisms in patients receiving diuretics provide a rational basis for the addition of drugs with renin or sympathetic inhibitory effects, which can produce marked additional decreases in blood pressure (Drayer et al, 1982c; Weber and Drayer, 1984). It is also of some interest that the therapeutic use of a low-sodium diet, which is probably analogous to diuretic therapy, can produce decreases in blood pressure in hypertensive patients but can also cause paradoxical pressor responses in a significant minority (Lund-Johansen, 1970). Presumably, these responses reflect the countervailing effects of renin and sympathetic stimulation.

In general, diuretics appear to temper exercise-induced blood pressure increases in hypertensive patients. During chronic diuretic therapy, this finding is probably due to the decreased total peripheral resistance and plasma volume and to a lesser degree of increase in cardiac output during the exercise (Lund-Johansen, 1970). However, it is possible that patients receiving high doses of diuretics in whom there is a marked decrease in plasma volume together with the neuroendocrine compensatory responses can actually experience an exaggerated increase in blood pressure with exercise (Ogilvie, 1976). An intrinsic problem with the hemodynamic picture during diuretic therapy is that the usual large increase in cardiac output during exercise is modified. Because an increase in cardiac output is vital in ensuring adequate transportation of oxygen and energy requirements to the exercising muscles and to the myocardium itself, especially during prolonged exercise, diuretic-treated patients tend to have a reduced exercise tolerance and a greater tendency toward exhaustion. Additionally, depletion of both sodium and potassium, which is a usual accompaniment of diuretic therapy, may hasten fatigue of muscle tissue. The plasma potassium concentration, which typically is reduced before the start of exercise, is subjected to two further influences during intense physical activity: the exercise itself, especially if large muscle groups are involved, can increase availability of potassium to the plasma by releasing it from the exercising muscles; on the other hand, the increased epinephrine produced during exercise, as described earlier, can drive potassium into cells and thereby worsen the preexisting tendency toward hypokalemia. It has been speculated that the unexpected high rate of cardiovascular mortality during some clinical trials of antihypertensive therapy might have been due to the antiarrhythmic impact of profound hypokalemia produced by the combined effects of diuretic therapy and physical stress (Hollifield, 1984).

β-Adrenergic Blocking Agents Although other classes of antihypertensive agents are rapidly growing in popularity as first-step therapy, the β-blockers remain as the most commonly used nondiuretic drugs for this indication. They are effective in decreasing blood pressure when used by themselves or in combination with diuretics or other agents. There are two groups of patients in whom the exercise properties of the β-blockers are interesting. The first group are young individuals in whom claims have been made that the β-blockers are more effective in lowering blood pressure than in the elderly. However, young people are more likely to engage in rigorous physical exercise and to be exposed to any potential negative impacts of β-blockers. The second interesting group of patients are those older individuals who have angina pectoris and for whom β-blockers are an effective treatment for their symptomatic ischemic heart disease as well as for hypertension. In these patients, the therapeutic properties of the β-blockers may actually help to improve exercise tolerance.

As with the diuretics, the initial hemodynamic response to the administration of β-blockers is not usually reflective of the long-term pattern. There is an immediate reduction in heart rate, stroke volume, and cardiac output, sometimes by as much as 25%, associated with an increase in total peripheral resistance (Dreslinski et al, 1982; Tarazi and Dustan, 1972). The blood pressure may decrease slightly or remain at its pretreatment level. After several hours or days of continuing β-blocker therapy, there is a tendency for the cardiac output to in-

Table II. **Effects of five weeks of treatment with β-blockers on total peripheral resistance index in hypertensive patients (from Tsukiyama et al, 1982, with permission).**

	Total peripheral resistant index		
Drug	Baseline	Treatment	Change
Control patients	2680 ± 128[a]	2752 ± 131	+2.7%
Acebutolol	2723 ± 94	2674 ± 157	−1.8%
Metoprolol	2724 ± 224	3000 ± 253	+10.1%
Propranolol	2078 ± 117	2617 ± 249	+25.9%[b]

[a]Values are mean ± SEM.
[b]p <0.05.

crease, although it still usually remains below its original baseline value; at the same time, the total peripheral resistance starts to fall, sometimes to its original pretreatment value or even slightly below. But even with long-term therapy, the total peripheral resistance tends to be somewhat greater than that in normotensive control patients (Tarazi and Dustan, 1972).

It is possible, too, that the total peripheral resistance during chronic β-blocker treatment may be a reflection of pharmacologic properties, such as cardioselectivity, of the differing individual agents. A comparison of the effects on total peripheral resistance of some commonly used β-blockers is given in Table II (Tsukiyama et al, 1982). These data show that after five weeks of active treatment, agents such as acebutolol, which have some partial agonist properties in addition to cardioselectivity, have no net effect on total peripheral resistance; metoprolol, which has cardioselective but not partial agonist properties, causes a modest 10% increase in total peripheral resistance; and propranolol, which is not cardioselective, produces a significant 25% increase. In direct measurements of forearm vascular hemodynamics (Levenson et al, 1984), it has also been shown that the long-acting hydrophilic β-blocker nadolol has virtually no effects on blood flow, whereas propranolol significantly increases vascular resistance. Interestingly, nadolol also has been shown to significantly decrease renal vascular resistance during chronic therapy (Frohlich et al, 1984; Hollenberg et al, 1979), a finding that has not been consistently reported with other β-blocking agents.

Studies with β-blockers in normal volunteers have indicated a reduction both in load and duration of dynamic exercise (Kaiser et al, 1986). Compared with placebo, both propranolol and metoprolol decrease heart rate and systolic blood pressure at maximal exercise (Sklar et al, 1982). It has been suggested that during dynamic exercise in normal subjects, the β-blockers do not appear to reduce blood flow to skeletal muscles. However, these types of studies have not yet been reported in patients with established hypertension in whom the resting hemodynamic profile, as well as the circulatory response to exercise challenges, may be different than those in normal subjects.

The β-adrenergic receptors found in vascular tissue are of the β_2 type and produce vasodilation when stimulated by substances possessing β-agonist properties. As discussed earlier, epinephrine appears to be released during dynamic exercise and to stimulate this β_2-mediated vasodilation, for in untreated normal individuals, the usual response to this type of exercise is a modest decrease in diastolic pressure despite the stimulatory effect of the catecholamines on the heart itself. In the presence of β-blockade, it could be theorized that the circulating catecholamines no longer get access to the vasodilatory vascular β-receptors and now produce an unopposed vasoconstriction through their actions on the arterial α-receptors (Epstein et al, 1965). Not surprisingly, it has been reported that dynamic exercise-induced increases in blood pressure appear to be less with cardioselective (β_1) blockers such as atenolol or metoprolol than with nonselective agents (Floras et al, 1983). However, there is actually great variability among individual patients in their blood pressure responses to exercise during β-blocker treatment (Hannson, 1975); indeed, regardless of the pharmacologic properties of the agent used, there is little evidence that exaggerated blood pressure responses occur (Hannson, 1975; Tarazi and Dustan, 1972).

All β-blockers appear to decrease heart rate and cardiac output responses to exercise, a factor that would be anticipated to decrease the maximum workload. As a practical matter, however, the majority of patients are sedentary in nature or are interested only in relatively modest degrees of exercise; in such patients, there is little evidence for any meaningful change in their routine work capacity (Frisk-Holmberg and Strom, 1986).

An important subgroup of patients with hypertension are those who concurrently have ischemic heart disease. In these patients, β-blockers are often very effective in treating the anginal symptoms. When these β-blocker-treated patients undertake either dynamic or isometric activity, the usual increases in cardiac output do not generally occur and changes in peripheral resistance are relatively minimal. This lack of hemodynamic reactivity is probably due to decreases in myocardial contractility as well as the β-blocker-induced decreases in heart rate. However, because the slower heart rate allows a prolongation of the diastolic filling period, with an improvement in coronary perfusion, exercise duration is actually increased. Moreover, the likelihood of anginal symptoms or of ST segment depression occurring during exercise is markedly reduced by β-blocker therapy (Ellestad, 1980). Thus, unlike normal volunteers, patients with ischemic heart disease can be improved to a significant extent by agents such as propranolol (Pratt et al, 1981).

The influence of β-blocking drugs on dynamic training in patients with ischemic heart disease is shown in Table III. In this study, it was found that an eight-week structured conditioning program of treadmill or bicycle ergometry in untreated

Table III. **Effects of training on exercise duration and workload in patients with ischemic heart disease in the presence or absence of β-blocker therapy (from Lowenthal and Kendrick, 1985, with permission).**

Parameter	Untreated		β-Adrenergic blocker treatment	
	Pretraining	Posttraining	Pretraining	Posttraining
Exercise duration (minutes)	10 ± 3[a]	14 ± 3	9 ± 3	14 ± 4
Exercise workload (kpm)	595 ± 313	1020 ± 375	474 ± 279	933 ± 337

[a]Values are mean $\pm$ SD; all changes from pretraining to posttraining are statistically significant.

patients with ischemic heart disease markedly increased exercise duration and almost doubled the exercise workload (Hare et al, 1984). Patients treated with β-blocking agents and subjected to the same dynamic conditioning program were found to have improvements in exercise performance that were identical to those observed in the untreated patients. Thus, although β-blockers may blunt or alter the normal hemodynamic responses to exercise, clearly they do not prevent the beneficial impact of a systematic conditioning program.

It is possible that pharmacologic characteristics of the β-blockers might influence the responses to dynamic exercise of patients with ischemic heart disease. It has been claimed, for example, that the decrease in cardiac output and the increase in pulmonary wedge pressure that occur in patients with coronary artery disease with propranolol were not seen when these patients exercised with either pindolol or labetalol (Silke et al, 1983). The partial β-agonist properties of pindolol and the presence of α-blocking properties (in addition to the β-blocking properties) of labetalol might have helped decrease peripheral resistance and cardiac afterload, thereby allowing improved cardiac performance during exercise. Additionally, cardiac output might have been better sustained in those patients treated with pindolol and labetalol because these agents are less likely than propranolol to cause bradycardia.

Isometric exercise can produce marked increases in both systolic and in diastolic blood pressures, and there has been theoretical concern that these effects may be heightened in the presence of β-blocker therapy. It has been demonstrated, however, in studies with the nonselective agent propranolol and the cardioselective agent atenolol that blood pressure at rest and during isometric exercise actually is reduced (Lowenthal et al, 1984b). In fact, the exercise-induced increment in blood pressure is the same during treatment as in the absence of treatment, but because the β-blockers decrease the resting blood pressure levels, the absolute values of blood pressure during exercise are now lower. An example of such a study is shown in Figure 3, summarizing an experience with propranolol and with labetalol (Weber et al, 1984). These observations, obtained during prolonged handgrip stimulation, show that neither drug increased or decreased the blood pressure reaction to the isometric exercise. Thus, the absolute values reached during this test were lower than the blood pressure found during an earlier placebo phase. These findings are similar to those observed by others (Virtanen et al, 1982) and indicate that hypertensive patients on β-blockers are unlikely to experience untoward effects with isometric stimuli. However, patients with impaired myocardial function, including early congestive heart failure, may experience dangerous increases in blood pressure if they are exposed to isometric stress during β-blocker therapy (Nelson et al, 1982).

A key factor in the response to exercise is an appropriate ventilatory increase. It has been found that ventilation and the exchange of oxygen and carbon dioxide are all decreased during submaximal workloads early in the course of propranolol treatment, although later the ventilatory response becomes more adequate (Tesch and Kaiser, 1983). It is possible that part of the problem may be a direct bronchoconstrictor action of β-blockers that inhibits the enhancement of airway function normally required by exercise. However, even in patients with chronic obstructive lung disease, the β-blockers do not appear to decrease the sensitivity of the ventilatory response to carbon dioxide during exercise (Leitch et al, 1980).

It could be conjectured that β-blockers might alter release of catecholamines from sympathetic nerve terminals in the peripheral circulation, thereby modifying pressor responses to sympathetic stimuli. Since the presynaptic β-receptors might have a regulatory influence on catecholamine release, treatment with β-blockers might decrease the amount of catecholamines transmitted. Overall, plasma norepinephrine concentrations during exercise do not change significantly during β-blocker treatment (Christensen and Brandsborg, 1973), perhaps reflecting the offsetting effects of the exercise itself and the possible inhibitory effects of the β-blockers on norepinephrine release.

When compared with placebo, nonselective β-blockers such as propranolol can increase plasma concentrations of potassium during dynamic exercise (Lowenthal et al, 1982a). This may be due, in part, to the inhibitory effect of β-blockers on the renin-aldosterone axis resulting in a tendency for renal potassium retention. A more important mechanism may be related to the epinephrine-mediated cellular potassium uptake during exercise. Because the entry of potassium into cells under these circumstances is regulated predominantly by β_2-adrenergic receptors (Weber et al, 1974), plasma potassium concentrations are likely to be higher in the presence of nonselective β-blockers than when cardioselective agents or placebo are administered.

The other metabolic effects of the β-blockers, however, might be of greater importance in determining responses to exercise. In patients with compromised coronary function, β-blockers appear to have a beneficial impact for they decrease oxygen demand. There is also a tendency for the myocardium during exercise to

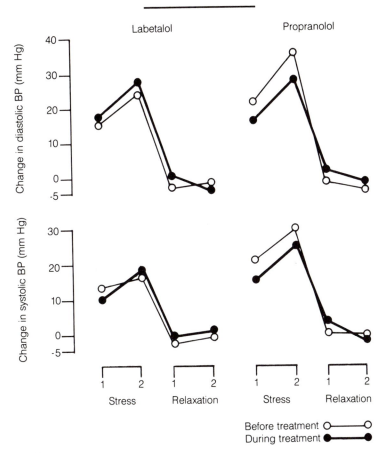

Figure 3.
Effects on systolic and diastolic blood pressures of isometric exercise (handgrip) before and during treatment of hypertension with labetalol or propranolol. Average values (n=15) are shown after one and two minutes of the stress and after one and two minutes of the subsequent relaxation (from Weber et al, 1984, with permission).

become more dependent on glucose as an energy source than on free fatty acids, which in turn may help to minimize ischemic damage in the zones of the myocardial tissue (Kurlen and Oliver, 1970; Ople, 1975). Unfortunately, the effects of β-blockers on skeletal muscle, both in uncomplicated hypertensive patients as well as in patients with ischemic heart disease, may be counterproductive. A first problem appears dependent upon local hemodynamics; not only is there some reduction in blood supply to muscles as a result of the reduced cardiac output caused by the β-blockers, but it is also possible that the relative vasoconstriction resulting from blockade of the peripheral vascular vasodilatory β_2-receptors might partly reduce skeletal muscle blood supply. Clearly, this could have an adverse effect on exercise endurance.

A second problem pertains to the effects of the β-blockers on local metabolism; the inhibition of phosphorylase produced by these agents prevents glycogen breakdown, a factor that also limits maximum exercise. Moreover, lactate translocation from exercising muscles into the blood is decreased during β-blocker treatment (Frisk-Holmberg et al, 1979), especially when nonselective agents are used (Frisk-Holmberg et al, 1981). It has been shown that blood concentrations of glucose, nonesterified fatty acid, and glycerol are all decreased during dynamic exercise in patients receiving agents such as propranolol or metoprolol; moreover, there are increases in glucogen concentrations, perhaps related to decreases in glycogenolysis in skeletal muscle (Lundborg et al, 1981).

Similar metabolic changes appear to be induced in the liver, for the β-blockers appear to reduce hepatic glycogenolysis during exercise (Newsholme, 1977). Moreover, exercise-induced lipolysis in fatty tissue is decreased by the β-blockers (Franz et al, 1983), thereby limiting the formation and availability of free fatty acids. This is of importance in individuals undertaking prolonged exercise, especially if the availability of glucose from glycogen stores has already been reduced. There do not appear to be major differences between selective and nonselective β-blockers in their effects on energy metabolism during exercise.

Overall, the effect of β-blockers on exercise performance is of interest because these agents appear to specifically block the epinephrine-mediated mechanisms that normally regulate the hemodynamic and metabolic responses to exercise. Although this effect is probably not of importance to individuals who engage in only modest levels of physical activity, β-blocker therapy is probably not acceptable to the majority of serious athletes. On the other hand, these agents can be of considerable help to the patient whose activity is limited by ischemic heart disease; in such individuals, the potential for improvements in coronary filling and for a reduction of symptoms can contribute to conditioning programs that can enhance exercise performance substantially.

Angiotensin Converting-enzyme Inhibitors   Early studies with captopril, the first clinically available converting-enzyme inhibitor, were based largely on patients with severe or treatment-resistant hypertension. More recently, it has been established that captopril, as well as other converting-enzyme inhibitors, is effective when used as first-line or single-agent therapy in a large proportion of patients with mild or moderate hypertension (Weber and Zusman, 1986). Moreover, captopril has been found to be effective over the broad demographic spectrum; it works in older patients as well as in the young and in black patients as well as in whites. The converting-enzyme inhibitors also are therapeutically effective in patients with congestive heart failure, and captopril is approved for this use.

In hypertensive patients studied at rest, the principal hemodynamic effect of captopril is a reduction of blood pressure associated with decreased total peripheral resistance (Cody et al, 1978; Heel et al, 1980). The cardiac output does not change substantially, although there have been some reports of a slight increase at rest (Fagard et al, 1980; Fujitani et al, 1979), perhaps consistent with the ability of this agent to improve cardiac function in patients with heart failure.

In patients with uncomplicated hypertension, however, cardiac function as reflected by ejection fraction remains constant during chronic therapy (Ventura et al, 1985). It is of some interest to directly evaluate the state of constriction of large arteries in the body for they have been shown to be partial determinants of cardiac afterload (O'Rourke, 1982) and also to contribute to the maintenance of hypertension (Gent, 1972). The use of techniques such as pulsed Doppler velocimetry for measuring blood flow and the slope of decline in arterial pressure during diastole as a measure of compliance when applied to the human brachial artery have indicated that captopril can directly produce vasodilatory effects in major vessels (Simon et al, 1985).

The decrease in total peripheral resistance with captopril is mirrored by similar changes in renal vascular resistance (Ando et al, 1986). It has also been shown that enalapril is able to decrease renal vascular resistance in uncomplicated hypertensive patients without altering renal function (Bauer, 1984). This property may separate the converting-enzyme inhibitors from other classes of vasodilators that do not produce the same degree of vasodilatation in the renal circulation as in the systemic circulation. It has also been noted in animal studies that captopril can shift the cerebral autoregulatory curve such that blood flow to the cerebral circulation is not impaired even in the presence of marked hypotensive responses (Barry et al, 1984).

Hemodynamic measurements obtained during exercise immediately following administration of captopril have shown a desirable pattern; there is an increase in cardiac output due chiefly to an increase in heart rate rather than in stroke volume, a decrease in total peripheral resistance, and a modest decrease in blood pressure (Fagard et al, 1982). During more chronic treatment with captopril, blood pressure responses to exercise have been variable. Some investigators reporting changes during treadmill exercise have indicated no change in either blood pressure or heart rate (Pickering et al, 1982), but others have found that exercise in captopril-treated patients causes modest decreases in both systolic and diastolic blood pressures (Manhem et al, 1981); indeed, it has been claimed that the decrease in blood pressure during exercise is greater than observed at rest (Fagard et al, 1982).

Hormonal measurements during exercise after several days of captopril therapy have indicated that angiotensin II and aldosterone, which are suppressed by captopril at rest, remain low during exercise. Moreover, there appear to be only minimal changes in plasma concentrations of norepinephrine and epinephrine (Manhem et al, 1981). These hemodynamic and hormonal responses to exercise in captopril-treated patients would indicate that there should be little if any impairment of exercise performance during this form of therapy. Indeed, it has been confirmed that exercise tolerance appears to be fully maintained during treatment with this converting-enzyme inhibitor (Heel et al, 1980).

α-Blockers and Vasodilators Prazosin, the prototype of selective α_1-blocking agents, has been the only α-blocking agent available for the treatment of hypertension, but other drugs in this class are expected to become available soon. In addition to their blood pressure-lowering properties, these agents also may have a beneficial impact on the cholesterol profile. At rest, chronic treatment with prazosin has been found to produce a desirable hemodynamic picture; blood pressure and total peripheral resistance are significantly reduced, and there is no change in cardiac index. During dynamic exercise, the cardiac output tends to increase, and there is a further fall in total peripheral resistance (Lund-Johansen, 1975). During rigorous arm and bicycle ergometry, there are some increases in heart rate and in blood pressure, but these changes are no greater than those observed with placebo administration (Lowenthal et al, 1984a).

During isometric stress, produced by handgrip, prazosin can decrease the peak exercise measurement for both diastolic and systolic blood pressures without producing any change in heart rate (Lowenthal et al, 1984b). Heart work, as measured by the product of the systolic blood pressure and the heart rate, might be slightly reduced, possibly an important factor in patients with underlying ischemic heart disease. Prazosin also appears to improve cardiac output during exercise in patients with borderline congestive heart failure.

The direct-acting vasodilators such as hydralazine or minoxidil decrease blood pressure at rest through reduction of total peripheral resistance but tend to increase both heart rate and cardiac output. This profile is opposite to that observed with the β-blockers and may be disadvantageous in patients with angina pectoris or other evidence for ischemic heart disease (Moyer, 1953). These agents, which tend to cause a greater degree of arteriolar dilatation than venous dilatation (DuCharme et al, 1973), can produce beneficial decreases in cardiac afterload in patients with congestive heart failure. But when used as antihypertensive agents, the vasodilators lose much of their efficacy through reflex sympathetic stimulation that increases cardiac output by stimulating both heart rate and myocardial contractility and also by increasing plasma renin activity (Gottlieb et al, 1972; Koch-Weser, 1974). During dynamic exercise in patients with uncomplicated hypertension, treatment with hydralazine does not impair the expected increase in stroke volume; moreover, in patients with congestive heart failure, hydralazine tends to further increase stroke volume and to decrease pulmonary wedge pressure during exercise (Ginks and Redwood, 1980). During isometric exercise, hydralazine does not appear to attenuate the stimulation of the sympathetic nervous system (Lowenthal et al, 1984b). Despite their vasodilatory properties, these agents do not appear to increase blood flow to skeletal muscles during exercise in patients with hypertension or with congestive heart failure (Koch-Weser, 1974; Wilson et al, 1981). Thus, if used as single-agent therapy, they do not appear to provide an ideal background to exercise.

Centrally Acting Agents The available centrally acting antihypertensive agents include methyldopa, clonidine, and guanabenz. The latter two drugs are very similar to each other in their pharmacologic effects. These agents work primarily through α_2-agonist actions in the central nervous system and produce a reduction in sympathetic outflow. During rest and exercise, these agents decrease plasma concentration of catecholamines (Virtanen et al, 1982). The principal hemodynamic effect of methyldopa in hypertensive patients at rest is to reduce both cardiac output and total peripheral resistance (Lund-Johansen, 1978a), although the major factor in its antihypertensive action is the reduction in total peripheral resistance (Safar et al, 1979). Clonidine produces similar changes in cardiac output and total peripheral resistance. The small reduction in cardiac output is not related to changes in myocardial contractility or in stroke volume but to a modest reduction in heart rate that results from a stimulatory effect of clonidine on vagal mechanisms. Renal blood flow is well maintained during clonidine treatment (Onesti, 1978).

During bicycle ergometry, methyldopa has been shown to modify exercise-induced increases in blood pressure and heart rate (Sannerstedt et al, 1962). The predominant effect of the methyldopa during exercise is on systolic blood pressure. Overall, effects on total peripheral resistance and cardiac output during exercise appear to be somewhat variable (Chamberlain and Howard, 1964; Lund-Johansen, 1972), although both parameters may decrease slightly. Clonidine also modifies the blood pressure response to exercise (Lowenthal et al, 1982a,b; Lund-Johansen, 1974) and possibly through its vagal effect might have a somewhat greater tendency than methyldopa to slow the heart rate during exercise as well as at rest. However, there is no evidence that cardiac output is reduced by clonidine during chronic treatment. The blood pressure responses to handgrip exercise are not altered by either methyldopa or clonidine (Lowenthal and Kendrick, 1985).

The usual endocrine responses to exercise, including hyperkalemia, and increases in plasma renin activity and aldosterone, are not greatly changed by either methyldopa or clonidine (Lowenthal et al, 1982a; Rosenthal et al, 1982), although the increase in plasma renin activity is somewhat blunted. Importantly, there is no evidence for any change in pulmonary function during exercise when the centrally acting agents are administered (Messerli et al, 1981a).

Calcium-channel Blockers The calcium-channel blockers have been found to be effective antihypertensive agents, especially in older patients. Like the β-blockers, they are effective treatment for angina pectoris and have been proposed as an ideal form of therapy in those patients who have concurrent hypertension and ischemic heart disease. Although the calcium-channel blockers might have some slight inhibitory effects on myocardial contractility, and especially on conduction, their principal effect in hypertension is to lower blood pressure through a reduction in total peripheral resistance (Lund-Johansen, 1984). These agents also appear to preserve renal blood flow and function (Loutzenhiser and Epstein, 1985). The three calcium-channel blockers now available, nifedipine, diltiazem, and verapamil, have each been shown to modify the maximum increase in blood pressure during dynamic exercise (Gould et al, 1982; Klein et al, 1983). Comparisons with β-blockers are of interest. It has been found that nifedipine is equivalent to metoprolol in its ability to modify the blood pressure response to exercise; if the two agents are given in combination, there is no further decrease in exercise-stimulated blood pressure effects (Ekelund, 1985). In another study comparing diltiazem with propranolol, it was found that both agents were more effective than placebo in attenuating exercise-induced diastolic blood pressure responses, but propranolol was more effective than diltiazem in preventing increases in systolic blood pressure and in heart rate (Yamakado et al, 1983). During chronic therapy, it seems that calcium-channel blockers might share with the β-blockers an inhibitory effect on exercise and optimal exercise performance. In patients undergoing several weeks of conditioning, increases in maximal ventilatory oxygen consumption and exercise time during treadmill testing were greater in patients receiving a placebo than in those receiving nifedipine (Duffy et al, 1984). If the nifedipine treatment was then stopped, subsequent testing indicated a significant improvement in performance. Thus, it is possible that calcium-channel blockers might partly limit the full beneficial effects of a conditioning program. Beyond their effects on the heart, it is possible that the calcium-channel blockers may modify conditioning and exercise performance by direct effects on skeletal muscle and on lactic acid metabolism (Halperin and Cubeddu, 1986).

In patients with ischemic heart disease, the calcium-channel blockers may be of benefit during exercise. There is a decrease both in myocardial oxygen demand and in afterload, resulting in a decrease in exercise-induced episodes of angina pectoris and in the likelihood of ST segment depression (Moskowitz et al, 1979; Subramanian et al, 1982). One further advantage of the calcium-channel blockers may be found during isometric exercise, where these agents have been shown to modify the stress-induced increases in blood pressure (Klein et al, 1983; Stein et al, 1984).

CONCLUSIONS

The chief characteristic of established hypertension is increased peripheral resistance, although a high cardiac output may play a role in some younger patients. Most of the modern classes of antihypertensive agents are effective in controlling hypertension at rest. During prolonged dynamic exercise, a clear increase in cardiac output should occur; systolic blood pressure should remain constant or fall. These hemodynamic adjustments provide increased blood supply to the exercising skeletal muscles and to the myocardium. Energy requirements are met by appropriate changes in glucose and lipid metabolism and by increases in ventilation. Antihypertensive drugs can influence these responses in differing ways.

Because epinephrine-like mechanisms mediate many of these exercise-induced changes through actions at β-adrenergic receptors, the β-blockers may decrease exercise load and duration. But in patients with ischemic heart disease, these agents may improve coronary perfusion and decrease anginal symptoms during exercise, thereby improving performance. The calcium-channel blockers similarly are of value in patients with ischemic heart disease. Diuretics may decrease exercise tolerance by modifying the needed increase in cardiac output and by causing sodium and potassium depletion. Centrally acting sympatholytic agents and α-adrenergic blockers do not appear to substantively alter exercise performance. Likewise, there are no adverse effects on physical activity during treatment with the converting-enzyme inhibitors. Although these issues do not appear to be critical in patients with sedentary lifestyles, it may be important to select an appropriate type of antihypertensive agent in individuals planning to undertake programs of exercise.

Chapter V

Quality of Life: An Important Consideration in Antihypertensive Therapy

Gordon A. Williams, MD,

and Marcia A. Testa, MPH, PhD

INTRODUCTION

The term quality of life has a variety of definitions because it probably does not represent a single measurable construct, such as blood pressure. Rather, this term is useful in organizing a variety of social and physical features of an individual's life. Primarily, it denotes an individual's ability to function in a number of different roles in society and to achieve a certain level of satisfaction from carrying out the activities associated with these roles.

Prior to the 1980s, concern about the quality of life of a hypertensive patient did not reach a high level of priority. Medical efforts were primarily directed at identifying the hypertensive patient and prolonging his or her life by reducing blood pressure with effective medications. During the 1970s and early 1980s, a variety of medications became available to treat hypertensive patients. Also, extensive public health campaigns uncovered the majority of patients who had hypertension.

With resolution of these problems, concerns about the impact of drug therapy on the patient's quality of life began to emerge. For example, two large-scale studies (Curb et al, 1985a; Medical Research Council [MRC] Working Party, 1981) reported substantial dropouts from clinical trials of patients treated for their hypertension. In most circumstances, the dropouts were secondary to adverse effects of the drugs on the patient's well-being. The adverse effect went beyond an increase in adverse physical symptoms also impairing the patient's ability to function effectively in a number of his or her roles in society. Thus, in a very real sense, the drugs were having a negative impact on the patient's quality of life.

The purpose of this chapter is to review the background of the development of the concept of quality of life and to address the application of this concept to the evaluation of drug therapy in the treatment of hypertensive patients.

EVOLUTION OF THE CONCEPT OF QUALITY OF LIFE

The Origins of the Concept   The concept of quality of life has been used in many different ways and for many diverse purposes (Campbell et al, 1976; Najman and Levine, 1981). Quality of life itself does not represent a single measurable construct but rather is useful as an organizing concept that encompasses the many emotional, psychological, and social indices of life quality (Figure 1). In the health care professions, the concept of quality of life has emerged largely from its roots in the social sciences. Used in the context of sociology, the term usually is employed to denote an individual's ability to function in a variety of social roles and to achieve a certain level of satisfaction from carrying out the activities associated with those roles.

The ever-increasing prevalence of chronic diseases has turned the focus of medical intervention from strictly curative to one that is preventative, with an emphasis on not only lengthening the life of the patient but improving the quality of life remaining (Frieds, 1980). In addition to physical limitations, individuals who are chronically ill encounter many social and psychological problems as a direct consequence of their disease. Studies relating changes in the quality of life resulting from the disease itself or the treatment of the disease are relatively limited. Most information concerning the emotional, social, and psychologic concomitants of disease and treatment tended to be anecdotal rather than experimental.

The prevention and management of a chronic disease frequently involves treatment regimens with negative influences on quality of life. Diseases such as cancer, rheumatoid arthritis, diabetes, hypertension, and chronic obstructive pulmonary disease often require administration of long-term and sometimes complex therapeutic regimens.

Any negatively perceived aspect of treatment beyond the disabilities associated with chronic disease can further restrict the patient's quality of life. The perceived efficacy of the treatment is often weighed against these negative aspects. For example, in the symptomatic patient with rheumatoid arthritis, the absence of pain resulting from the administration of steroids may be perceived positively when compared to the occasional gastrointestinal upset associated with this therapy. However, to the asymptomatic hypertensive patient, the same degree of gastrointestinal discomfort may be unacceptable. As such, the evaluation of treatment regimens upon the patient's quality of life must account for the individual characteristics of the patient's illness and the patient's perceptions of the treatment benefits.

In order to evaluate the full impact of the treatment of a chronic disease upon the total health status of the patient, biomedical researchers turned to the disciplines of social and behavioral sciences and adopted the concepts and theories concerning the evaluation of life quality. In addition to its sociological origins, the public health origins of the quality of life concept were derived not from economic and social therapy but from public health practices concerned with improving the environmental, educational, and preventative aspects of health care on an interdisciplinary basis. Chronic disease epidemiologists have not only

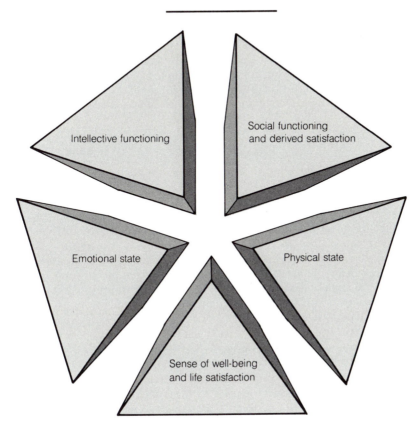

Figure 1.
The dimensions of the quality of life.
In order to assess any changes in a patient's quality of life during the 24-week study on antihypertensive therapy, Croog et al (1986) defined quality of life as consisting of five components: sense of well-being, physical state, emotional state, intellective functioning, and social functioning.

documented the risk factors associated with disease prevalence but have also studied widely their impact upon life quality.

During the early 1970s, the adoption of this concept by medical care professionals was documented during a series of Congresses sponsored by the American Medical Association on improving quality of life. During this period:

> "... the American Medical Association (AMA) dedicated itself to improving the quality of life in the bicentennial years and thereafter. In sponsoring the series of Congresses on Improving the Quality of Life (in the Early Years, 1972; in the Middle Years, 1973; and in the Later Years, 1974),

the AMA has elected to serve as an organizational catalyst to increase public awareness of the need for, and the wisdom of, attacking our sociological, environmental, educational, and medical problems on an interdisciplinary basis. . . . We are encouraged by the number of quality of life programs that are being promoted . . . . There is no purpose more important than a dedicated effort to improve the quality of life in America as our heritage to the generations to be born in the third century of our nation."

John H. Budd, MD
Program Chairman
AMA Congress III
(Brown and Ellis, 1975)

Indices of functional disability are being used increasingly to rate the status of patients studied in clinical research or treated in clinical practice during the eighties (Feinstein et al, 1986). In response to this growing trend, Feinstein coined the term "clinimetric" to describe an index used as a rating scale for symptoms, clinical conditions, and other clinical phenomena. His reviews (Feinstein, 1982; Feinstein et al, 1985) of more than 1000 such indices indicate the large interest that has emerged in attempting to quantify varying degrees of disease disability, including functional, occupational, social, and emotional aspects of the patient's quality of life.

QUALITY OF LIFE AND ANTIHYPERTENSIVE THERAPY

Assessment of the efficacy and incidence of adverse reactions associated with antihypertensive therapy has been the primary focus of clinical trials designed to monitor the impact of therapy on the hypertensive patient. However, with an increasing emphasis on preventative medicine and the long-term treatment of mild to moderate hypertension, examination of the impact of therapy in terms of the psychological and social dimensions of living (ie, the patient's quality of life) is becoming increasingly important to both scientific investigators and practicing clinicians involved with the treatment of hypertension.

Quality of Life and Compliance in the Hypertensive Patient   One of the reasons for the increased awareness and emphasis on the evaluation of antihypertensive therapy and life quality has to do with patient compliance. Presently, the major factor limiting effective treatment of patients with hypertension is noncompliance (Haynes et al, 1982). This applies regardless of whether they are involved in pharmacologic or nonpharmacologic treatment programs. The reasons underlying this noncompliance are not entirely understood. In part, however, they may be related to the patient's perception that 1) he or she is asymptomatic, and 2) most, if not all, antihypertensive agents are likely to produce long-term side effects (Curb et al, 1985b; Nies, 1975).

The extent of this problem can be appreciated by noting the withdrawal rates in large clinical trials involving hypertensive patients. The British MRC trial, which enlisted thousands of patients with total treatment years now exceeding 60,000, has an overall withdrawal rate of 20% to 25% (MRC Working Party, 1981). A withdrawal rate of greater than 30% was reported by the Hypertension Detection and

Table I.   Adverse reactions of antihypertensive medications.

Class	Common adverse reactions
Diuretics	
Thiazide-type	Hypokalemia, hyperuricemia, hyperglycemia, hyponatremia, hypercalcemia, hyperlipidemia, rashes, other allergic reactions
Loop	Hypokalemia, dehydration, hypocalcemia, hyperuricemia, metabolic alkalosis, rashes
Potassium-sparing	Hyperkalemia, gastrointestinal disturbances, gynecomastia (spironolactone), rashes
β-Adrenergic blocking agents	
Acebutolol Atenolol Metoprolol Nadololol Propranolol Timolol	Fatigue, bradycardia, congestive heart failure, bronchospasm, Raynaud's phenomenon, depression, sleep disturbances, gastrointestinal disturbances
Peripheral sympatholytic agents	
Reserpine	Depression, nightmares, drowsiness, gastrointestinal disturbances
Guanethidine	Orthostatic hypotension, fluid retention, bradycardia, diarrhea
Prazosin	Dizziness, drowsiness, fatigue, syncope, fluid retention
Central sympatholytic agents	
Methyldopa	Sedation, dizziness, bradycardia, orthostatic hypotension, gastrointestinal and liver disorders, Coombs' positive hemolytic anemia
Clonidine	Dry mouth, drowsiness, sedation, sleep disturbances, rebound hypertension upon withdrawal
Arteriolar dilating agents	
Hydralazine	Gastrointestinal disturbances, tachycardia, aggravation of angina pectoris, lupus-like syndrome
Minoxidil	Hypertrichosis, fluid retention, tachycardia, pericardial effusions
Angiotensin converting-enzyme inhibitors	
Captopril Enalapril	Rash, dysgeusia

Follow-up Program after five years (Curb et al, 1985a). The patients participating in both of these studies were treated with conventional therapy, for example, diuretics, reserpine, β-blockers, and methyldopa. In the nontrial, clinical practice setting, the lack of adherence to the prescribed program is even more immediate and dramatic. Sackett and associates (1975) describe data indicating that approximately 50% of patients discontinued taking their antihypertensive medication after only six months.

The impact of therapy upon the patient's quality of life is likely to be a main determinant in the patient's ability to comply with the prescribed treatment regimen and to continue with antihypertensive therapy. If the patient's perceived "gain" in terms of blood pressure control and reduced risk of cardiovascular disease is much less than the "loss" due to the side effects of medication, the potential for continuing on antihypertensive therapy is minimized. Furthermore, when these side effects are manifested in ways other than the commonly cited and easily observed adverse reactions and physical symptoms, such as extreme fatigue, impotence, headache, dry mouth, dizziness, nausea, and bradycardia, both patient and physician might remain unaware of the impact of the antihypertensive therapy upon the patient's total well-being. The need for increased awareness has been summarized by Light (1980), who states " . . . there is a very great need to document the behavioral side effects associated with specific antihypertensive agents so that these considerations may be weighed along with other factors when the physician chooses the best prescription and dosage for each patient."

The reported adverse reactions that have been associated with the use of different classes of antihypertensive medications are listed in Table I. Recent efforts to address the problem of noncompliance have focused on producing agents that have fewer adverse reactions and physical side effects as well as developing techniques to quantify psychological, social, and behavioral side effects. In order to monitor these less clinically apparent side effects of antihypertensive therapy and their association with the patient's quality of life for both clinical research and practice, it is first necessary to define and measure quality of life in substantive terms. The following section will define the concept of quality of life so that it can be applied to the quantitative assessment of quality of life in the mild to moderately hypertensive patient during active therapy.

84

ASSESSING QUALITY OF LIFE IN THE HYPERTENSIVE PATIENT

Definition of Quality of Life Mild to moderate hypertension is generally asymptomatic and, as such, the patient generally feels well. Traditionally, the goal of antihypertensive therapy has been to prevent future complications, such as stroke, coronary heart disease, congestive heart failure, and kidney failure, and not necessarily to make the patient feel better. Measurement of the total impact of antihypertensive therapy can be accomplished through careful monitoring of the patient's quality of life, which encompasses the biomedical, behavioral, and social dimensions of living.

Recently, medical research studies and clinical trials have included quality of life measures as principally dependent variables that must be scientifically analyzed to gain a rigorous, comprehensive, and complete understanding of therapeutic interventions. The scope of medically based quality of life measurement is quite broad and has been assessed in many different ways for different target populations (Bergner et al, 1976; Breslow, 1972; Grogono and Woodgate, 1971; Hill et al, 1985; Kaplan et al, 1979; Katz and Akpom, 1976; Meenan et al, 1980; Robertson, 1985; Sackett et al, 1977; Westaby et al, 1979).

Table II. **Assessment techniques required to clinically monitor the many levels of quality of life (adapted from Testa, 1987a, with permission).**

Component	Assessment technique	Measures
Presence of adverse reactions and physical symptoms	Clinical exam	Simple checklist of common reactions
Distress associated with symptoms	Preclinical questionnaire	Physical, sexual, somatic, cognitive
Emotional status	Preclinical questionnaire	Well-being, vitality anxiety, depression, sleep disturbance
Life satisfaction	Preclinical questionnaire or interview	Social, personal, marital, job,

The various methods for assessing quality of life range from the measurement of functional status in the terminally ill to the emotional and social status of patients with less limiting diseases. While the quality of life of the terminally ill and severely disabled patient can usually be measured in terms of functional status, measurement of quality of life in patients with mild to moderate hypertension with minimal or no physical impairment is much more complex. In fact, the complexity of the measurement is simply a function of the many facets of life that the treated but seemingly healthy hypertensive patient is able to experience.

A report by Furberg and colleagues (1984) on defining quality of life in the mildly hypertensive patient concluded that quality of life should be defined by its various components. These components fall into three broad categories, namely, functions, perceptions, and symptoms. More specifically, functions were defined in terms of one's personal, social (work, family, friends), emotional (distress, well-being), and intellectual (alertness, memory) states. The other two categories included the patient's perception of life satisfaction and health status as well as subjective and objective measures of symptoms.

A similar approach to defining quality of life in the hypertensive patient was proposed by Levine and Croog (1984), who defined quality of life in terms of five underlying dimensions, namely 1) the sense of well-being and satisfaction with life, 2) the physical state, 3) the emotional state, 4) cognitive processes, and 5) the ability to perform in social roles and the degrees of satisfaction derived from those roles. The restrictions to these dimensions is selective, and yet they are considered crucial components of life quality in most industrialized societies.

For hypertensive patients, quality of life is best defined in terms of the major components of life quality for the healthy individual. Many of the measures used to assess these components are highly correlated and mutually dependent. If one's goal is to monitor the effects of therapy, concentrating on those components most immediately affected by the therapeutic intervention is probably the most practical. From a clinical perspective, a hierarchical approach to the definition of quality of life is useful (Testa, 1987a). This approach layers the various measures according to how easily they can be observed during the course of a clinical examination (Table II). Each successive layer (Figure 2) requires a more complex assessment by the clinician in order to obtain information on associated changes in the different areas of quality of life relating to the prescribed regimen. Indeed, a sudden change in satisfaction with one's marriage or job may be mediated through concomitant changes in affect, libido, vitality, concentration, or sense of well-being. Such alterations may be directly or indirectly related to distress caused by side effects of medication. The possible connection between a patient's remark, such as "I don't feel I'm able to cope with the stress of my job," and increased lethargy caused by a therapeutic agent is often overlooked.

Common physical symptoms (extreme fatigue, loss of taste, nausea, headache, dizziness) can be assessed objectively and are most immediately apparent to the patient. The patient's subjective perceptions and degree of distress related to other less clinically apparent symptoms (change in sexual functioning, perceived physical changes) form the second layer. The third layer involves the patient's emotional (distress, well-being) and intellectual (alertness, memory) states. Finally, the patient's degree of satisfaction with life, which is largely affected by the three previous layers, forms the inner core.

Assessment of Quality of Life: Psychometric Techniques Measurement of quality of life in the hypertensive patient comprises assessment of a set of variables that extend beyond the usual biomedical indices associated with health. It is an organizing concept that brings together dimensions of physical, emotional, social, and intellectual capabilities, perceptions, and functions. Each of these areas can be divided into subcomponents that can be measured through psychometric testing procedures. Many standardized tests for the assessment of symptoms, emotional status, well-being, and life satisfaction are currently available. Assembling these measurement instruments under the organizing concept of quality of life is the primary requirement for measuring the less clinically recognizable side effects of antihypertensive medication. The result is a battery of tests and questions relating to the patient's functions, perceptions, and distress with symptoms.

By combining results from the clinical history and examination with a series of self-assessment questionnaires on functions and degree of life satisfaction, it is possible to monitor changes in the treated hypertensive patient that can impact upon the patient's acceptance of therapy. The hierarchical approach to the assessment of quality of life during the clinical examination involves psychologically "invasive" procedures requiring a more in-depth analysis of the patient's functions and perceptions than is usually undertaken during the typical clinical examination. The most practical approach to such evaluation is through patient self-assessment questionnaires and interviews with a spouse or close relative.

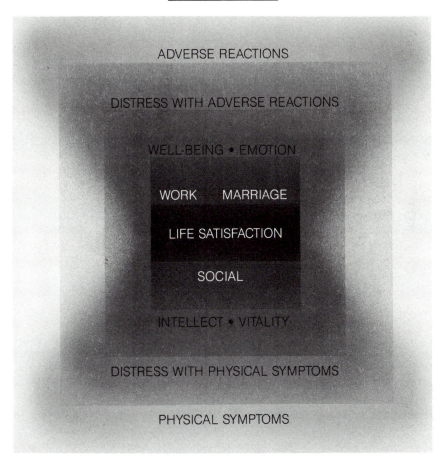

Figure 2.
Assessment of quality of life requires probing more deeply than in the typical physical exam — beyond the assessment of physical side effects to factors such as symptom distress, well-being, emotional state, intellect, vitality, and the patient's satisfaction with his or her life roles.

Selection of the appropriate measures for the assessment of quality of life components usually involves combining existing measurement instruments into a battery of tests administered to the patient within a single session. For the hypertensive patients, these tests should involve measurement of the following areas.

Measurement of Symptoms   The patient's general health and functional status are objective conditions that can have a considerable effect on the patient's quality of life, especially when there are acute changes that have a negative impact on the patient's physical state. In the seemingly healthy hypertensive patient, these acute changes often manifest themselves as physical side effects of medication. In addition to the presence of clinically observable physical symptoms, the patient's tolerance of physical impairments is an important component in assessing quality of life. A new physical symptom, such as dry mouth, while minor when compared to the progressive symptoms of pain and loss of mobility in the rheumatoid patient, may have the same degree of impact on the patient's perception of life quality. Therefore, in addition to recording the presence or absence of adverse reactions, the degree of distress associated with such symptoms is also important.

The recording of adverse reactions should be part of the clinical history. In addition, the patient can be asked to rate the degree of distress (none, somewhat, moderate, quite a bit, extreme) related to a list of symptoms, such as dizziness, loss of taste, inability to concentrate, weakness in body parts, and problems in sexual functioning. The Symptom Check List (SCL-90; Deragotis and Spencer, 1982) is useful for psychologically based symptomatology not directly cited as a typical side effect of antihypertensive therapy. Given that the patient might not freely admit to distress associated with particular symptoms or even to the symptoms itself, an independent assessment from a spouse or close relative is often useful for further validation.

Measurement of Functions   The patient's sense of well-being in terms of ability to function is a subjective measure of life quality that individuals can report relative to their own life experiences. Sense of well-being also can be divided into subcomponents, including measures of satisfaction with one's general health, personal life, work, and daily activities; measures of positive indices, such as vitality, happiness, cheerfulness, enthusiasm, as well as the degree of negative indices, such as fatigue, anxiety, and depression. These measures capture the internal rating scale of each individual patient rather than objectively assessing the scope and breadth of activities the patient experiences.

The concept of the patient's sense of well-being, an internally scaled dimension, is an extremely crucial component to the assessment of life quality. All questions are framed such that the patient judges the degree of vitality, cheerfulness, depression, and anxiety relative to his own experiences. Measurement instruments useful for this include the General Well-Being Schedule (Dupuy, 1973) or an adaptation of it, for example, the Mental Health Inventory (Veit and Ware, 1983) or the Profile of Mood State (McNeir et al, 1971). Once again, objective assessment by a spouse or other close relative can add further information on the degree or actual level of positive or negative aspects of well-being independent from the patient's responses.

Measurement of Satisfaction   The conventional usage of the term "satisfaction" refers to the complete fulfillment of a need or want and the attainment of a desired end (*Webster's Third New International Dictionary*, 1981). The term has been used in psychological testing to refer to an assessment of the overall conditions of existence as derived from the comparison of one's aspirations to one's actual achievements. It would appear that, by definition, the degree of life satisfaction as measured by the degree of personal fulfillment derived from one's personal, social, and family roles is a much more stable construct than either symptomatology or functions. Certainly, acute changes in life satisfaction due to antihypertensive therapy are probably more closely linked to alterations in physical and emotional status and the chronic adjustment to such alterations.

Examples of tests that measure life satisfaction include the Kutner Morale Scale (Kutner et al, 1956), the Life Satisfaction Index-A (Neugarten et al, 1961), the Self-Anchoring Scale (Cantril, 1965), and the Philadelphia Geriatric Center Morale Scale (Lawton, 1972).

Assessing the Impact of Medical Intervention on Quality of Life The type of medical intervention that is selected can affect the patient's life quality. For example, a dramatic negative change in life quality can be experienced when a patient requires treatment that can have a profound impact upon the patient's ability to perform individual and social roles, such as is seen with routine dialysis or chemotherapy. Alternatively, positive changes and an improved quality of life are often reported in patients undergoing reconstructive surgery for correction of a severe disability. The risk of surgical complications with the potential for reducing quality of life has always been a primary consideration in the decision of whether or not to perform elective surgery that could potentially improve life quality.

89

The comparative measurement of two or more treatments with regard to quality of life considerations has been quite evident in decisions concerning therapeutic surgical interventions. For example, in the case of a patient with breast cancer, the decision to perform a radical mastectomy or a simple mastectomy with radiation therapy involves both considerations of expected survival as well as the resulting quality of life of the patient after surgery. Simple mastectomy, the less debilitating of the two, is thought to interfere less with the patient's ability to perform personal and social roles and to result in lower levels of anxiety, depression, and distress.

Comparison of the impact of lifelong treatment upon the patient's quality of life has also been of interest in the treatment of Type I diabetes. Conventional insulin therapy and continuous subcutaneous insulin infusion (CSII) therapy have been compared not only in terms of degree of glucose control but also in regard to the greater freedom and more satisfying lifestyle CSII therapy might offer the patient (Pickup et al, 1985).

Long-term pharmacologic interventions have always been assessed in terms of their potential toxic effects and incidence of adverse reactions. Pharmacologic agents that are efficacious and have low levels of adverse reactions are considered optimal therapy. Comparative trials of such agents usually involve assessing the difference in the incidence of adverse reactions and side effects between two equally efficacious therapies. Extending such comparisons to include both objective and subjective parameters of life quality has been proposed particularly in reference to antihypertensive medications (Williams, 1987).

A COMPARATIVE TRIAL OF ANTIHYPERTENSIVE THERAPY AND QUALITY OF LIFE

Design Factors   In addition to the standard requirements for a large-scale clinical trial, such as double-blindedness, randomization, accurate endpoints, and adherence to treatment protocol, four major issues should be addressed in the design of a study to evaluate the effect of therapy on the quality of life of the hypertensive patient. These include the sensitivity of the measurement instrument, the impact of the diagnosis, the effect of the doctor/patient relationship, and the social, economic, and demographic characteristics of the study population. The ability of the quality of life index to measure change is an extremely important factor in detecting a treatment effect in a clinical trial (Testa, 1987b). While many indices are useful for purposes of discrimination or prediction, only evaluative indices that measure the magnitude of longitudinal change are effective in the detection of a treatment differential in a clinical trial.

Several research studies have documented that simply labeling a patient as hypertensive has a negative effect. For example, Haynes and colleagues (1978) screened for hypertension in the workplace. The patients, first told they had hypertension at the time of screening, had a fivefold increase in absenteeism due to illness in the year following the screening, as compared with the previous year

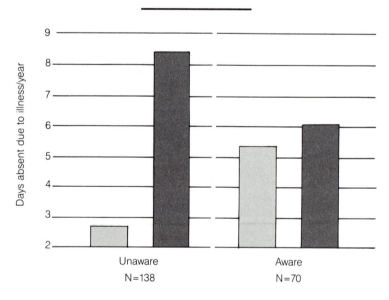

Figure 3.
Work absenteeism in the year before ( ) and after (■) labeling of hypertensive patients. Two hundred and eight subjects formed the basis of this study; 138 were previously unaware, and 70 previously aware that they had hypertension (adapted from Haynes et al, 1978, with permission).

Table III.   Impact of antihypertensive therapy on quality of life (assessed in general practice; from Jachuck et al, 1982, with permission).

Assessment by: Outcome	Physician	Patient (Percent reporting) N = 74	Relatives
Improved	100	48	1
No change	0	43	0
Worse	0	9	99

(Figure 3). Thus, in any study designed to assess the effect of drug therapy on quality of life factors, one needs to consider the impact of labeling.

Changes in the patient's health status can be viewed from many different perspectives. Often, the terms improvement or worsening following treatment can be interpreted at many different levels. For the physician, improvement might mean only reduction in blood pressure while to the patient it might mean reduction in blood pressure with no other negative effects of medication. Moreover, relatives of the patient might consider only the impact of the therapy on the patient's life quality. The extent of this phenomenon has been most dramatically documented by Jachuck et al (1982). They selected 74 hypertensive subjects and asked them, their spouses, and their physicians whether normalizing blood pressure with drugs had led to an improvement, a worsening, or no change in the patient's quality of life. The treating physicians nearly all responded that the patient's life was improved. However, only about 50% of the patients agreed with their physicians. Most surprising was the response of the relatives of the hypertensive patients. It was their perception that, even though the blood pressure was lowered, the patient was actually worse on therapy than prior to its initiation (Table III). The implications of these results are twofold: 1) any measurement should be based upon a prospective assessment of specific measures of quality of life not subject to differences in interpretation, and 2) quality of life must be accepted as a construct that contains both objective and subjective parameters with inherent responder variability.

The level of blood pressure itself may affect the quality of life. Bulpitt et al (1976) studied the effect of standard hypertensive therapy (diuretics, reserpine, methyldopa, and β-blockers) on several quality of life factors in hypertensive patients matched for sex and age to normotensive subjects and untreated hypertensive patients. All three groups were drawn from a clinic population. Of particular interest, however, was the increase in side effects observed in the untreated hypertensive patients when compared with the normotensive control group (Figure 4).

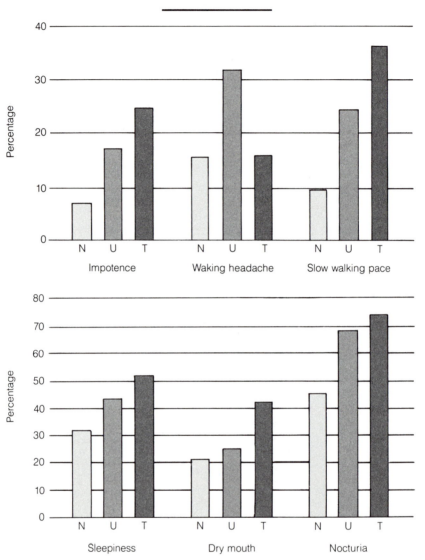

Figure 4.
Complaints in normotensive (N), untreated (U), and treated (T) hypertensive patients. All patients were drawn from a general medical clinic: 78 normal subjects, 99 untreated hypertensives, and 477 treated hypertensive patients (adapted from Bulpitt et al, 1976, with permission).

For all parameters except dry mouth, the untreated hypertensive patients had a significantly greater frequency of side effects than did the normotensive. Thus, this study strongly suggests that consideration needs to be given to the level of blood pressure at the time the quality of life factors are assessed.

Additionally, the design of a quality of life study must take into account the definition of "a good life" in the population under investigation. For example, women and men or the employed and unemployed may have quite different perceptions of what an adverse effect is. This perception may manifest itself in several ways: it is likely that questions designed to assess depression in unemployed individuals, for example, may be less sensitive than individuals who are employed simply because an unemployed state usually leads to a relatively greater degree of depression. Thus, a drug causing depression may have little adverse impact in an unemployed individual. Alternatively, a drug that improves depression may actually have a more beneficial effect in an unemployed individual than in an employed individual where little further improvement may be possible. On the other hand, individuals working in a highly competitive field may have a higher level of anxiety than those working in less competitive fields. Under these circumstances, drugs that lower blood pressure and also reduce anxiety would be more beneficial in the former than in the latter individual. Thus, depending both on the characteristics of the drugs used and the population studied, results of clinical trials assessing the impact of treatment on the quality of life might vary considerably.

Quality of Life Clinical Trial

Study design Based on the above considerations, an ideal clinical trial to evaluate the effects of antihypertensive therapy on quality of life factors should be measured against the following goals: 1) normalization of blood pressure; 2) a single daily drug dose is preferable to multiple daily dosing because of the difficulty of relating dose effects to quality of life data; 3) the quality of life questionnaire should not be administered by a physician but by someone who is specifically trained to carry out the interview in an objective fashion; and 4) in order to reduce the inherent "noise" in the assessment, these studies are best carried out in a homogeneous population in terms of gender and cultural, ethnic, and social backgrounds. The obvious corollary to the design of such a clinical trial is that information should be extrapolated to other populations only with extreme care.

Many of the aforementioned desirable features were incorporated into a recent clinical trial that compared the effect of captopril, methyldopa, and propranolol on several quality of life factors (Croog et al, 1986). This study used a homogeneous population consisting of white employed males between the ages of 21 and 65 who had mild to moderate hypertension (diastolic blood pressure between 92 mm Hg to 109 mm Hg on three determinations).

Patients with a history of allergy, drug hypersensitivity, recurrent dermatoses or collagen disease, presence of significant gastrointestinal disease, renal insufficiency, neutropenia, myocardial infarction within two years, history of cerebrovascular accident, severe mitral or aortic valvular disease, medical contraindications to any of the three study drugs, or use of psychotropic drugs during the two weeks prior to the entry into the study were excluded from the recruitment procedure.

A total of 761 patients were recruited for the study, and after a four-week placebo washout period, 626 entered the double-blind active treatment phase. The most common reasons for exclusion from the treatment phase included blood pressure levels that were too high or too low to meet the study protocol, lost to follow-up, perceived adverse reactions to placebo, and poor compliance with the drug regimen.

The primary goal of the study was to test the ability of psychometric techniques to detect differences in the effects of antihypertensive therapy on quality of life. Methyldopa, a drug that commonly produces adverse effects, was administered in a dose of 500 mg twice daily as a positive control, and captopril, a converting-enzyme inhibitor that has been reported to have minimal side effects, was administered in a dose of 50 mg twice daily as a negative control. These two agents were compared with propranolol 80 mg twice daily, a standard antihypertensive agent. Hydrochlorothiazide 25 mg twice daily was added to all these regimens if blood pressure could not be normalized by monotherapy after the initial eight weeks of treatment.

Patients were interviewed and surveyed for quality of life baseline and change measures at entry, 8 weeks, and 24 weeks after treatment by registered nurses or medical administrative and technical health personnel who were not directly associated with the care of the patients. All interviewers received standardized training.

The assessment of quality of life included incidence of withdrawal due to adverse reactions, distress due to perceived physical side effects, development or exacerbation of sleep dysfunction, measures of well-being, emotional status, social participation, life satisfaction, visual memory and psychomotor function, and work performance and satisfaction.

Results

Study population characteristics The average age of the patient population was 48 years, weight 93 kg, systolic blood pressure 145.6 mm Hg, and diastolic blood pressure 97.8 mm Hg. Overall, the group was highly educated (an average of at least two years of college), employed largely in executive/professional or small business/managerial positions, mostly married (80%), and in the upper 50th percentile for income. Approximately 74% of patients had received previous antihypertensive medication before entering the study. No significant differences were found among the three treatment groups with regard to demographic, clinical, or quality of life measures.

Control of blood pressure was comparable in all three groups at the end of 24 weeks. The mean 24-week diastolic blood pressure levels were 87.1 mm Hg, 87.7 mm Hg, and 86.1 mm Hg, respectively, for patients treated with captopril, methyldopa, and propranolol. Use of a diuretic was more prevalent at 24 weeks for patients treated with captopril (33%) than for methyldopa (28%; p = not significant versus captopril) and propranolol (22%; p <0.02 versus captopril).

Changes in quality of life during treatment Analysis of the quality of life data was directed at two major questions: 1) do patients improve, worsen, or remain stable during treatment when compared with baseline levels, and 2) was there a difference in the pattern of change among the three treatment groups?

Figure 5 shows the withdrawal rates due to adverse reactions for the three treatment groups. Patients on captopril withdrew significantly less often (8%; 17 pa-

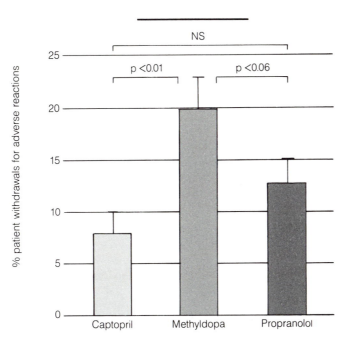

Figure 5.
Percent of patients who withdrew from active therapy because of adverse drug effects (adapted from Croog et al, 1986, with permission).

tients) when compared with methyldopa (20%; 39). The withdrawal rate for propranolol was 13% (27 patients). The most common adverse reaction was fatigue or lethargy, with 21 reactions reported in the methyldopa groups, 15 in the propranolol, and 6 in the captopril group. Other reasons for withdrawal are given in Table IV.

Captopril produced positive and statistically significant changes for the quality of life measures of well-being, physical symptoms, sexual functioning, work performance, sleep dysfunction, cognitive skills, life satisfaction, and social participation. In comparison, treatment with methyldopa resulted in significant worsening for measures of physical symptoms, sexual functioning, work performance, and life satisfaction. Propranolol showed worsening in physical symptoms, sexual functioning, and life satisfaction (Figure 6).

Comparisons of the pattern of change during treatment showed significantly more favorable changes for captopril as compared with methyldopa for the summary scores of general well-being and its associated subscales—anxiety, positive well-being, general health, and vitality. Captopril also showed more favorable changes with regard to physical symptoms, work performance, life satisfaction, and cognitive skills (Figure 7). In comparison with propranolol, patients on captopril showed significantly more positive changes in overall general well-being (and its associated components of positive well-being and vitality), physical symptoms, and sexual functioning. Scores for propranolol showed more favorable changes in work performance when compared to those on methyldopa (Figure 7).

This clinical trial has now undergone extensive secondary analysis with several additional publications (Croog et al, 1987; Testa, 1987b; Williams, 1987). The results of the trial have been analyzed in terms of its impact on a typical clinical practice (Testa, 1987b). With the treatment differential observed in this study for well-being between captopril and methyldopa (with or without a diuretic), the physician could expect to see twice as many patients with substantial worsening treated with methyldopa as opposed to captopril. In patient numbers, 20% of patients treated with methyldopa and 15% of patients treated with propranolol could have been spared worsening in their general well-being if they had been treated with captopril.

All secondary analysis of primary data should be interpreted with caution. One of the more intriguing observations is what appears to be a negative impact of diuretic therapy upon quality of life (Figure 8). Those individuals who required a diuretic in order to normalize blood pressure had a substantial worsening of their overall general well-being index, which was particularly noteworthy for

Table IV. **Adverse drug reactions associated with withdrawal from the quality of life clinical trial, according to number of occurrences reported[a] (from Croog et al, 1986, with permission).**

	Treatment group[b]			
Adverse reaction	Captopril (N = 17)	Methyldopa (N = 39)	Propranolol (N = 27)	Total (N = 83)
Fatigue, lethargy	6	21	15	42
Sexual disorder	5	6	6	17
Sleep disorder, nightmares	2	5	2	9
Headache	2	5	2	9
Dry mouth	0	6	2	8
Dizziness	0	5	3	8
Nausea	0	4	2	6
Bradycardia	0	0	6	6
Myalgia, muscle cramps	0	3	1	4
Anxiety, irritability	3	0	1	4
Palpitations	2	1	0	3

[a]The reactions listed are those that occurred among patients who withdrew from the study and that were reported by three or more patients.
[b]There was a total of 30 adverse reactions in the captopril group, 89 in the methyldopa group, and 51 in the propranolol group.

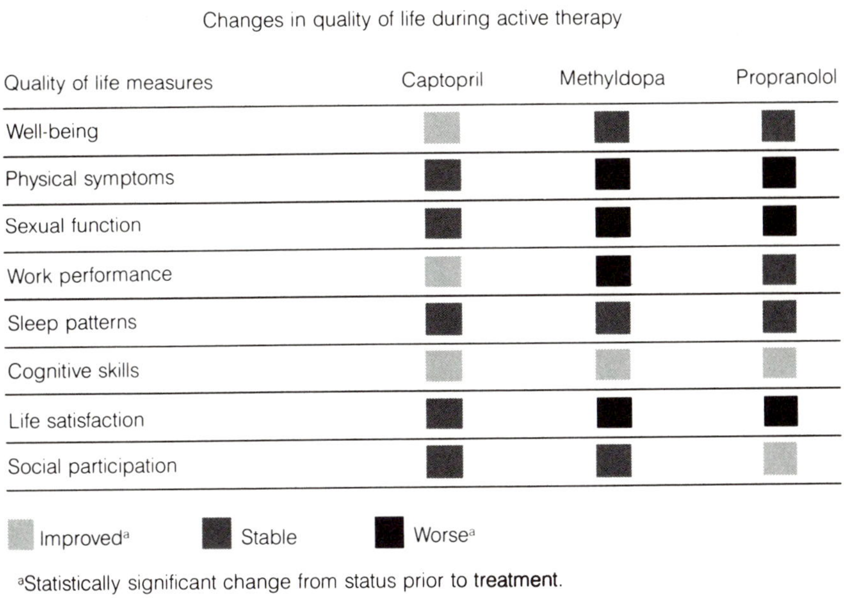

Changes in quality of life during active therapy

Quality of life measures	Captopril	Methyldopa	Propranolol
Well-being	Improved	Stable	Stable
Physical symptoms	Stable	Stable	Stable
Sexual function	Stable	Stable	Stable
Work performance	Improved	Stable	Stable
Sleep patterns	Stable	Stable	Stable
Cognitive skills	Improved	Improved	Improved
Life satisfaction	Stable	Stable	Stable
Social participation	Stable	Stable	Improved

▨ Improved[a]   ■ Stable   ■ Worse[a]

[a]Statistically significant change from status prior to treatment.

Figure 6.
The chart shows statistically significant changes in quality of life within each treatment group compared with a baseline measure. Patients taking captopril improved in general well-being, work performance, and cognitive skills and remained stable in all other measures. Patients taking methyldopa improved in cognitive skills, worsened in the scales for physical symptoms, sexual function, work performance, and life satisfaction, and remained stable in the other measures. The propranolol group improved in cognitive skills and social participation, worsened in physical symptoms, sexual function, and life satisfaction, and remained stable in the other measures (adapted from Croog et al, 1986, with permission).

propranolol and captopril. Captopril-treated patients requiring a diuretic had no net change in their general well-being index in contrast to what occurred in propranolol-treated patients who needed a diuretic for adequate blood pressure control. Captopril alone had a highly positive effect on the general well-being index. Indeed, the positive effect of captopril was as great as the negative effect of diuretics, propranolol, and/or methyldopa (Figure 8). Thus, in this clinical trial, captopril was not a negative control as originally assumed but demonstrated changes in quality of life consistent with a positive effect.

Finally, how extensively can the results of this clinical trial be extrapolated to other doses of the present drugs or other antihypertensive agents? One simplis-

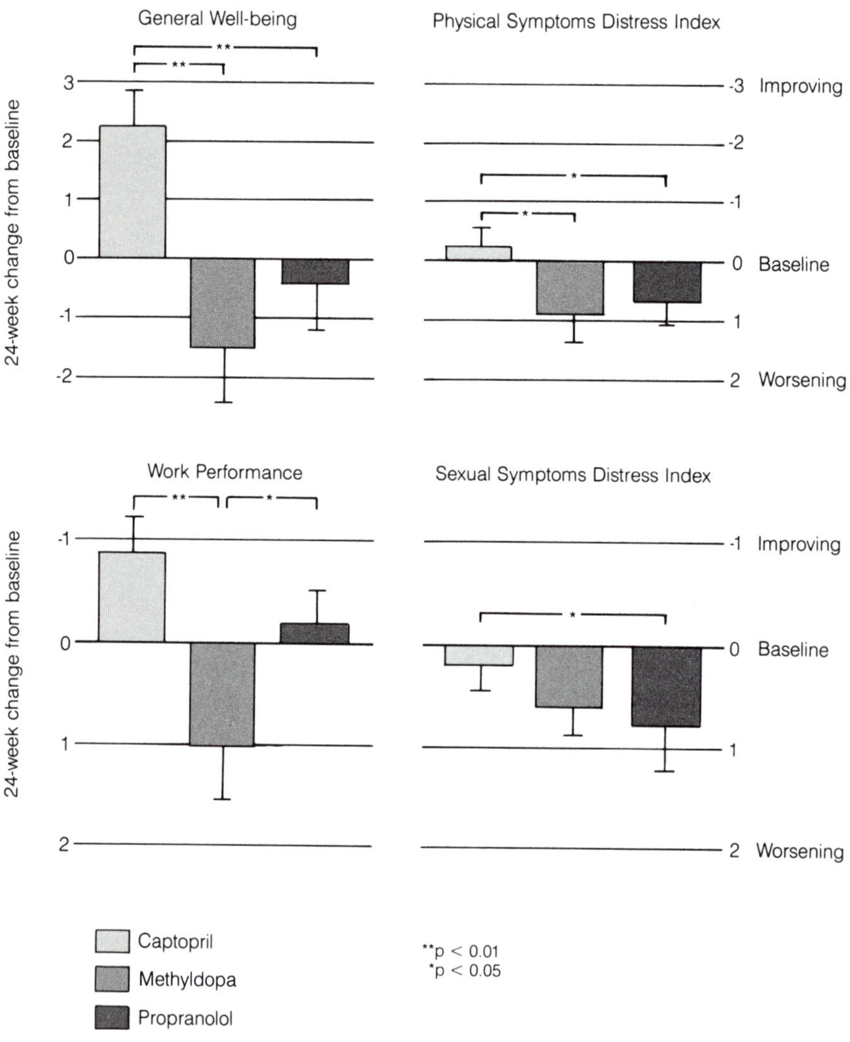

Figure 7.
Comparison of mean SEM rates of change 24 weeks from baseline for quality of life measures among the three treatment groups; * p <0.05, ** p <0.01 (adapted from Croog et al, 1986, with permission).

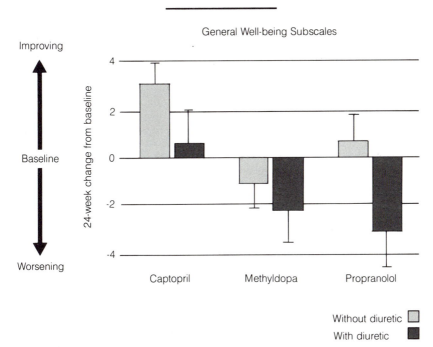

General Well-being Subscales

Figure 8.
Comparison of mean (±SEM) changes 24 weeks after therapy was initiated for general-well-being indices among the three treatment groups divided into those who received monotherapy and those requiring a diuretic. The number of patients in each subgroup were as follows: captopril (n=106), with diuretic (n=75); methyldopa (n=89), with diuretic (n=55); propranolol (n=117), with diuretic (n=49) (adapted from Williams et al, 1987, with permission).

tic possibility, for example, is that any agent that is free of central nervous system side effects (ie, a converting-enzyme inhibitor) will not have a negative impact on the patient's quality of life and indeed might improve his or her quality of life. Unfortunately, there is limited information available to verify this conclusion. The one other study performed examining the quality of life of patients treated with a converting-enzyme inhibitor (enalapril) does not agree with this assumption (Dahlof et al, 1985). In this study patients were withdrawn from antihypertensive therapy for a month and then placed on enalapril. Diuretic could be added to therapy if blood pressure control was unsatisfactory on monotherapy alone. Scores of quality of life improved when patients were changed from their previous therapy to placebo and showed no change (negative or positive) by subsequent treatment with enalapril.

Even though the two studies cannot be compared due to methodological differences, their results support the possibility that not all agents free of central nervous system side effects will improve quality of life of the hypertensive patient, but some will show only a neutral effect. Thus, it remains to be shown whether other agents lacking central nervous system side effects will have a neutral or positive influence on the quality of life of the hypertensive patient. Whether other β-blockers will have a response similar to propranolol is also uncertain. Theoretically, one might assume that the less lipophilic β-blockers would have fewer adverse effects. However, until specific studies are completed to document this, such conclusions appear unwarranted extrapolation of the presently available data.

Implications of Quality of Life Considerations for Antihypertensive Drug Selection The management of hypertension has undergone significant improvement and modification over the past several decades. Antihypertensive therapy has been shown to effectively reduce the risk of mortality and morbidity from congestive heart failure, stroke, renal disease, and other diseases associated with hypertension. Treatment of mild hypertension is now recognized as an accepted practice in the prevention of cardiovascular disease. As a consequence of the acceptance of treatment of mild hypertension, many more patients are undergoing antihypertensive therapy than ever before.

Accompanying the increase in the number of patients who are candidates for antihypertensive therapy are a number of new and improved agents that offer potential benefits over traditional therapy. The nature of these benefits appears to be derived from differences in side-effect profiles that lead to improved patient acceptance. Recent evidence indicates that the quality of life of the patient is a very important consideration in the selection of an antihypertensive therapy. Furthermore, there is now scientific evidence that antihypertensive agents do differ in their influence on quality of life measures. In this regard, captopril has been shown to offer some benefits over traditional antihypertensive therapy. Thus, clinicians must become aware of the impact of therapeutic intervention on the quality of the patient's life and apply this knowledge to their selection of antihypertensive therapy.

Chapter VI

Patient Population as Consideration for Antihypertensive Therapy

David B. Case, MD

INTRODUCTION

Perhaps the most important strategic change in the treatment of hypertension in the past few years has been an attempt to treat the hypertensive patient with medication that takes into account such factors as age, sex, race, and particularly other medical conditions, medications, and personal needs. These clinical factors are the most accessible to the practicing physician and need to be considered before initiating drug treatment. It would be ideal if drug therapy were also mechanism-specific; that is, if the drugs selected were specific and balanced counter regulatory mechanisms, such as renin secretion, sympathetic adrenergic tone, and renal sodium retention. Because this is not entirely possible or practical at this time, it must wait as a future development.

How patients with hypertension should be treated with drugs has been a subject of considerable debate in the past decade. In the era when it first became established that pharmacologic reduction of blood pressure reduced the occurrence of end-organ complications, there were only a few drugs to choose from, including diuretics and reserpine. As more agents emerged in the classes of sympatholytics, direct vasodilators, ganglioplegics, and others, the selection of a drug by the treating physician was based more on his experience than a scientifically devised strategy. However, most of the original antihypertensive drugs, such as reserpine, pargyline, and guanethidine, are seldom used anymore as initial or even additive therapy because of their adverse side-effect profiles.

Because of the availability of many new, better-tolerated, and improved antihypertensive agents, a strategy for drug treatment of hypertension can now be based on a consideration of each patient's own available medical information. This information is readily accessible to the treating physician and usually does not include any sophisticated tests. The strategy takes into account what has been learned about the different therapeutic effects and side effects of the many recently developed medications. Of particular importance is the consideration of how various coexisting medical conditions and their drug treatments influence the selection of therapy for hypertension. This chapter will focus on individualization of drug therapy to specific patient populations.

REAPPRAISAL OF STEPPED-CARE

The National High Blood Pressure Detection and Follow-up Program (HDFP) led to the reappraisal of the strategy for treatment of hypertension (The Joint National Committee, 1984). The original recommendation to use diuretics as the initial therapy in all cases was based on the widespread use of thiazides, their effectiveness in lowering blood pressure, and their general acceptability. In addition, at the time, it accorded with the popular hypothesis that excess sodium chloride was in some way responsible for most hypertension. The results of the HDFP study provided further evidence that some of the risks of even mild hypertension in causing cardiovascular end-organ disease could be reduced by effective, diuretic-based antihypertensive regimens. However successful the study, a number of important questions were raised by the results:

1. Would the same outcome have occurred if drugs other than thiazide diuretics had been used first? In other words, did this uniform strategy provide more or less benefit than an alternate one that based the selection of drug therapy on the individual clinical and physiologic characteristics of each patient? Dollery (1985), for example, has recently demonstrated markedly different "benefit profiles" based on overall outcome in patients subgrouped according to age, race, sex, obesity, and underlying disease by comparing treatment with thiazide diuretics and β-blockers. Would there have been greater compliance had there been individually tailored treatment for each patient?

2. Do any of the medications used for treatment of hypertension provide benefit or protection to the target organs that is independent of their mechanism for reducing blood pressure?

3. Why was there so little apparent benefit in reducing the occurrence of myocardial infarction despite adequate blood pressure control?

4. Why did the initial recommended formula approach ignore the consideration of coexisting disease and concomitant drug use as major determinants of agent selection or exclusion? These considerations are particularly relevant in elderly patients.

These and other questions have led to a serious reappraisal of the so-called "stepped-care" approach for treating hypertension, which is based on the HDFP protocol. As a result, the authors of the HDFP have, for example, revised their recommendations to include commencing therapy with a β-blocker in certain cases (The Joint National Committee, 1984).

Currently, there has been an increasing trend to abandon the stepped-care approach in favor of individualized therapy, recognizing that the understanding of hypertension and the availability of many new drugs have provided new opportunities for treatment strategies. This does not deny, however, the value of the early systematized approach to treatment but rather recognizes the importance of including the latest thinking and pharmacologic advances into the current practice of medicine.

AGE AS A FACTOR IN SELECTION OF THERAPY

Standard antihypertensive therapy was designed with the usual patient being a middle-aged adult. There is now, however, substantial evidence that a fraction of children, adolescents, young adults, and particularly older or elderly individuals have levels of systolic and diastolic hypertension that require drug treatment. For both the younger and older hypertensive patients, there are special considerations that address their differences in physiology, drug metabolism, and coexisting needs and conditions.

Considerations for Both Younger and Older Hypertensive Patients At the extremes of age (ie, children and the elderly), attention has been called to increased potential for drug sensitivity, reduced drug clearance, and the possibility of paradoxical responses. As a general consideration, therefore, it has become a prudent practice to initiate therapy of any kind in reduced dosage in these subgroups. The dose may be increased incrementally until a therapeutic effect is obtained or a reasonable standard dose is achieved. If the response to therapy is inadequate with a standard dose, the possibility of a secondary form of hypertension, such as renovascular disease, should be considered. The relative frequency of renovascular hypertension is greater in the young and older populations, as compared to the general adult population in which essential hypertension predominates. By the same reasoning, an inadequate antihypertensive response to diuretic therapy coupled with the development of significant hypokalemia may also signal secondary hypertension (Hunt et al, 1974). A profound or exaggerated response to treatment with a converting-enzyme inhibitor, on the other hand, also suggests the possibility of underlying renovascular hypertension because these drugs block the formation of excess angiotensin II generated from renal ischemia (Case et al, 1982).

103

Considerations for the Young Hypertension in children and in young adults is frequently but not invariably characterized by increased sympathetic adrenergic activity, as reflected in higher plasma norepinephrine levels (Goldstein, 1981), increased cardiac output, and increased plasma renin activity (Hofman et al, 1981). Thus, the most specific agents to antagonize the typical pathophysiology are the antirenin or anti adrenergic drugs. Because extracellular fluid volume is usually normal or decreased in this age population, diuretic treatment would have less rationale. Agents of choice include converting-enzyme inhibitors, β-blockers, combined α-β-blockers, and α-blockers.

Angiotensin converting-enzyme (ACE) inhibitors are effective antihypertensive agents in both mild and severe forms of hypertension in childhood and adolescence, as has been demonstrated with captopril (Oberfield et al, 1979).[*] Because plasma renin levels are normal or elevated in most children and young adults, this class of drugs is likely to be effective in a substantial proportion of this group. ACE inhibitors do not diminish cardiac output and therefore do not impede athletic or physical performance. In addition, they may be administered in once-daily or twice-daily dosage and do not appear to interfere with mental or sexual-function. Because this class of drugs is relatively new, there is no long-term experience in large numbers of children or young adults to assess potential adverse or beneficial consequences.

[*]Squibb Editorial Note: Please refer to the full prescribing information regarding Pediatric Use and recommended dosage in pediatric patients.

β-Blockers reduce increased heart rate frequently found in young hypertensives as well as diminish plasma renin levels (Bühler et al, 1972). As a consequence, this class of drugs has proved to be particularly successful in controlling hypertension in children and young adults. Because most young adults have normal hearts and normal or increased cardiac function at rest, the reduction of cardiac output associated with β-blockers has minimal consequences for nonexertional conditions. For competitive athletes, however, chronic β-blockade reduces cardiac output by 15% at rest and by even a greater percent during maximal exertion (Tarazi and Dustan, 1976). This critical gap in cardiac performance may make the difference in competition. Such therapy may deservedly be resented by the aspiring athlete, particularly when there are alternative effective drugs, such as converting-enzyme inhibitors, which do not impair cardiac performance. Moreover, β-blockers may induce or exacerbate cold-induced asthma, a factor contrary to top performance in outdoor cool or cold weather sports. There have been a number of reports of sexual dysfunction during β-blockade, but there has been no information whether this affects younger hypertensives. Another consideration in young people is what the long-term consequences of β-blockade might be. Although the experience with β-blockers in hypertension is only a little more than a decade, there is no evidence to suggest that long-term treatment entails unforeseen adverse effects.

α-Blockers, particularly central α-agonists, have been used for many years to treat hypertension in the young. Although effective in reducing pressure, centrally acting agents have been observed to produce drowsiness, lethargy, sexual impotence, and depression. For these reasons and with the availability of many acceptable alternatives, these agents have fallen from favor. Prazosin, a peripheral acting $α_1$-antagonist, has been used in children with some success. This agent, however, requires two or more doses daily and therefore may produce problems with compliance. Terazosin, a longer acting $α_1$-blocker, may be preferred for this reason but has not been tested widely in young people. Some degree of postural hypotension is associated with $α_1$-blockers, which might interfere with a number of physical or athletic activities.

The combined α-β-blocker, labetalol, has some theoretical potential value in the hypertension of children and young adults because it combines peripheral α-blockade with only minimal β-blockade. For this reason, the drug tends to interfere less with maximal cardiac performance than standard β-blockers. Sexual impotence and interference with mental function have not been cited as significant side effects of either peripheral α-blockers or α-β-blockers.

Calcium-channel blockers have gained use for the treatment of hypertension in adults largely because of their concurrent use in the treatment of angina. Verapamil and diltiazem reduce cardiac contractility and heart rate, usually to a lesser degree than β-blockers. In contrast, nifedipine has only a minimal effect on these parameters (Spivack et al, 1983). All of these calcium-channel blockers are relatively short acting, that is, they last about six hours, requiring multiple daily doses. However, a sustained-release form of verapamil has recently been released, and a slow gastrointestinal-release form of nifedipine is in development, as are new long-acting calcium-channel blockers. One final consideration is cost: treatment with these agents is relatively expensive compared with alternative regimens.

Table I. Characteristics of elderly hypertensive population that require consideration in management.

- Greater tendency to develop glucose intolerance
- Carotid and aortic baroreceptor dysfunction
- Deterioration in mental function
- ↓ Plasma renin levels
- ↓ Renal function
- Tendency to constipation
- Limited medical care budgets

CONSIDERATIONS FOR ANTIHYPERTENSIVE TREATMENT IN THE ELDERLY

The older or elderly hypertensive patient must be approached with a somewhat different therapeutic strategy than the young or average adult patient. The chief reason is the likelihood of coexisting conditions, such as cardiac, vascular, or renal disease. In the evaluation of the older hypertensive patient, care must be taken to assess even the most subtle signs and symptoms of early congestive heart failure, angina, cerebrovascular disease (eg, bruits), and peripheral vascular disease. The priority of therapy is to treat hypertension with medication that does not aggravate any underlying condition. Ideally, this medication might treat or at least be compatible with other medical conditions. Some important characteristics of the older—in contrast to the average young adult—hypertensive patient are listed in Table I and are summarized here.

The elderly have a tendency to develop glucose intolerance when given thiazide diuretic treatment (Kohner et al, 1971). Measures to assess this include detailed information of family history, observations of blood glucose values over time, and, if thiazides are used, interval measurements of blood glucose or glycosylated hemoglobin.

Carotid and aortic baroreceptor dysfunction may be present in the elderly due to atherosclerosis. This dysfunction produces increased lability of pressure from reduced "buffering" by baroreceptors and increased vulnerability to postural hypotension. Before treatment in patients with marked variability of office blood pressures, it may be valuable to monitor 24-hour ambulatory pressure to determine the constancy of hypertension and its time course during the day. Treatment of patients with baroreceptor dysfunction should avoid agents with the potential for producing postural reductions in pressure, such as α-blockers and gangioplegic agents.

Gradual deterioration of mental function—memory, mood stability, alertness—may occur in the elderly. Drugs to be avoided are ones with central nervous system side effects that aggravate these variables. Central α-agonists, rauwolfia-reserpine compounds, and, to a lesser degree, β-blockers may affect mental functioning to a significant extent in the elderly. In contrast, diuretics, converting-enzyme inhibitors, and calcium-channel blockers are relatively neutral in this regard.

The elderly also have reduced plasma renin levels and functioning renal mass. Beginning in the seventh decade, there is a gradual decline in plasma renin levels in normal people and perhaps even more in patients with essential hypertension. This may reflect nephrosclerosis and diminished excretory capacity for sodium and chloride. Reduced renin levels indicate a lesser role for angiotensin in maintaining arterial pressure and, therefore, a potentially smaller response to single-drug therapy with drugs that lower blood pressure in part by acting on the renin system eg, (converting-enzyme inhibitors). The net impact of these age-related changes is the need for sodium restriction or diuretic therapy, in order to remove excess salt and to stimulate the renin system; this in turn facilitates treatment with agents that block the renin-angiotensin-aldosterone system.

A common functional problem of the elderly is constipation. Verapamil and to a lesser extent diltiazem produce or aggravate constipation, presumably by their action to relax bowel smooth muscle. Diuretics by producing a relative dehydration may also adversely affect bowel function by producing hard or inspissated stools. Thiazide diuretics, moreover, may induce hypokalemia and therefore slow bowel activity. In contrast, β-blockers by increasing vagal tone may enhance peristaltic action and thereby facilitate bowel motility.

COST AS A CONSIDERATION IN THERAPY

A current dilemma facing physicians prescribing antihypertensive medications is how to select the theoretical "best choice" of drug therapy when one agent may be very costly in comparison to other agents that may be less medically specific yet more easily affordable. The span of expense for treatment is great, ranging from as little as a few dollars per month for a generic thiazide diuretic to several hundred dollars for two or three newly developed drugs. The problem mirrors in a microcosm the inequities in the American health care system that are ultimately based on the ability to pay. Therefore, in the group of hypertensive patients with limited funds for drugs, it may be possible to justify as "best practical fit" the relatively inexpensive drugs, such as those that are available in generic form: thiazide diuretics, propranolol, methyldopa, hydralazine, their combinations, and others.

At the other end of the spectrum are the more expensive agents, such as calcium-channel blockers followed by converting-enzyme inhibitors, newer β- blockers and α-blockers, combination thiazide diuretic with potassium-sparing diuretic, or adrenergic blockers.

Because compliance for people with limited means may be related to the cost, the effectiveness of a treatment program can possibly be enhanced by a discussion of cost before initiation of therapy. If the responsiveness of the blood pressure makes this approach possible, it may provide the patient the opportunity to revise his therapy according to his financial circumstances. It may take a trial of inexpensive therapy that proves unsuccessful to justify the greater expense of the newer, "leading edge" medications.

In patients in whom cost of therapy is not a major consideration, however, compliance may be improved by initial selection of specifically tailored therapy with a priority for convenience and lack of side effects. Such products include combination drugs and the more recently developed long-acting drugs.

In summary, while cost of therapy should not in the best of circumstances be a deterrent to an open "best fit" selection, it must be considered in the poor, elderly on fixed income, and those primarily concerned with cost-containment.

COEXISTING DISEASE AND CONDITIONS THAT INFLUENCE ANTIHYPERTENSIVE THERAPY

In the middle-aged adult and the older hypertensive patient, the presence of coexisting chronic cardiovascular or other medical disease becomes an increasingly prominent consideration in the selection of individualized antihypertensive therapy. The following discussion will consider the more common coexisting conditions and describe how the various agents may interact with the condition and its usual treatment.

Central Nervous System Diseases and Conditions

Manic-depressive disorders A number of the older antihypertensive agents have been known to cause or aggravate depression. Included in this group are reserpine and the centrally acting α-agonists, such as methyldopa, clonidine, and guanabenz. Also included in this group are lipid soluble β-blockers, such as propranolol and metoprolol. On the other hand, for manic states and sympathetic overdrive conditions, such as drug withdrawal, propranolol and clonidine have proven to be therapeutic because of their sympathetic blocking properties.

107

Because the usual treatment of manic-depressive illness includes tricyclic or similar antidepressants and lithium salts, selection of antihypertensive therapy should consider the possible interaction with certain drugs. Tricyclic antidepressants produce postural hypotension regularly; therefore, reserpine, direct vasodilators, and α-blockers are not preferred treatment because they may potentiate this effect. On the other hand, converting-enzyme inhibitors do not affect postural regulation of blood pressure and may have subtle mood elevating activity (Cohen et al, 1984; Zubenko and Nixon, 1984). Although diuretics do not affect mood disorders directly, they reduce renal clearance of lithium and increase the risk of lithium toxicity and should be used with caution (Hurtig and Dyson, 1974). Methyldopa, aside from aggravating depression, may be ineffective when given with a tricyclic antidepressant (White, 1965), an effect presumably shared by other methyldopa-like drugs. Calcium-channel blockers appear to be relatively free from adverse interactions with mood elevating drugs, although little has been reported about drug interactions.

Psychotic disorders Several major antihypertensive agents may induce or aggravate thought disorders or interact with the usual treatment. Lipid-soluble β-blockers, such as propranolol, affect the central nervous system and may in a few predisposed but otherwise "normal" patients produce an organic brain syndrome or toxic psychosis; hallucinations, confusion, paranoia, agitation, suicide attempts, and nightmares have also been reported following β-blockers (Greenblatt and Koch-Weser, 1973; Shopsin et al, 1975; Stephen, 1966; Yorkston et al, 1976). When propranolol was used in high doses to treat schizophrenia in clinical studies, blood pressure actually rose significantly, to severe levels in some patients. Therefore, patients treated with lipid-soluble β-blockers should be followed closely to determine if psychiatric changes occur.

As a central α-agonist, methyldopa may produce a paradoxical rise in blood pressure when administered with phenothiazines and may increase the toxicity of haloperidol (Westervelt and Atuk, 1974). Because the drugs used to treat psychotic disorders eg, (phenothiazines) have significant α-blocking action of their own, antiadrenergic drugs may not be needed. Moreover, the use of peripheral α-blockers would seem redundant. Potentially useful drugs in patients with psychotic disorders include diuretics, ACE inhibitors, and calcium-channel blockers, all of which reduce blood pressure without adversely affecting thought disorders nor interfering with the usual antipsychotic drugs.

Other central system disorders Patients with migraine headaches may obtain relief from β-blockers, particularly those with lipid solubility, such as propranolol. Parkinson's disease is often treated with L-dopa, which is incompatible with methyldopa and possibly other central α-agonists.

Patients with cerebrovascular insufficiency should avoid drugs and combinations that produce postural hypotension. Therefore, direct vasodilators, reserpine-like drugs, and α-blockers should be used with caution. Diuretic treatment increases whole blood viscosity, which in turn might impair microcirculatory flow in the brain. This suggests the need to prevent excessive sodium depletion in patients already on diuretics.

108

TREATMENT OF HYPERTENSION AND COEXISTING CARDIAC DISORDERS AND EXERCISE NEEDS

A substantial fraction of hypertensive patients has some cardiac disease or condition. In addition, an increasing number of individuals with uncomplicated hypertension without cardiac disease exercise vigorously for fitness or recreation and do not want to have their peak athletic performance impaired by medication. A number of antihypertensive drugs, however, do reduce resting and/or exercise-induced increases in cardiac output. The following discussion will suggest preferred antihypertensive drugs for these cardiac-related conditions.

ANGINA PECTORIS

Angina is treated by improving nutrient myocardial blood flow and/or decreasing myocardial oxygen demand. Most antihypertensive drugs can potentially improve or at least not worsen angina because they reduce myocardial work, related to the product of systolic pressure x heart rate, and thereby oxygen demand without disproportionate lowering of myocardial blood flow.

β-Blockers and calcium-channel blockers are widely used to treat angina as well as hypertension. β-Blockers reduce heart rate and act to relieve angina by decreasing myocardial oxygen demand, especially during exercise (Frishman, 1981; Wolfson et al, 1966). These actions are particularly relevant in the hypertensive patient with angina who may exhibit an increased resting and exercise heart rate and a characteristic overshoot in arterial pressure with exercise. Both β-blockers and calcium-channel blockers attenuate myocardial contractility. β-Blockers have little effect on the coronary blood supply to ischemic myocardium, although there is a redistribution of blood flow to the subendocardial area (O'Rourke, 1985). In contrast, calcium-channel blockers produce coronary artery dilatation. In a review comparing these agents in hypertension, calcium-channel blockers were equally or possibly more effective in controlling angina than β-blockers, depending on the patient population studied and the doses used (O'Rourke, 1985).

Central α-agonists such as methyldopa have been used in patients with angina for many years, but there are no reports of direct benefit to the coronary symptoms. Methyldopa, as an example, reduces peripheral resistance and produces variable and small reductions in heart rate and cardiac index (Lund-Johansen, 1972). Cardiac contractility, however, estimated by left ventricular ejection time and time for preejection period, appears to decline (Karatzas and Clouva, 1979). Peripheral acting α₁-blockers possess similar hemodynamic characteristics as central α-agonists, and, thus, prazosin does not produce reductions in heart rate or cardiac output and does not have specific antianginal activity (Koshy et al, 1977).

The use of a direct vasodilator such as hydralazine by itself increases cardiac output and heart rate and may aggravate angina (Koch-Weser, 1974). Addition of a β-blocker will usually block those unwanted effects (Pettinger and Keeton, 1959).

ARRHYTHMIA

109

Arrhythmias may be caused or aggravated by increased ischemia. This may result from abrupt hypotension as can occur, for example, with the initial dose of prazosin. Supraventricular tachyarrhythmias have been observed to occur in hypertensive patients with otherwise intact baroreflexes during treatment with the direct vasodilators hydralazine and minoxidil (Koch-Weser, 1974). These effects may be reduced or blocked with concomitant use of a β-blocker.

Arrhythmias may arise from metabolic origins, chiefly from the depletion of potassium and, in association, magnesium. There has been considerable concern over the risk of hypokalemia-induced arrhythmias as a consequence of thiazide diuretic therapy (Freis, 1986; Stewart et al, 1985). Generally, it is agreed that levels of serum potassium should be maintained in the normal range by the use of concomitant treatment with potassium-sparing diuretics, potassium salt supplements, or ACE inhibitors. Angiotensin converting-enzyme inhibitors reduce aldosterone-induced potassium loss by blocking angiotensin II formation, resulting in a net gain of potassium (Atlas et al, 1979). The particular relevance of potassium conservation, as it relates to heart disease in general, is emphasized by the results of the European Working Party trial (Amery et al, 1985). In contrast to former studies using thiazide-based treatment not correcting serum potassium, this study showed that a thiazide combined with a potassium-sparing diuretic reduced mortality in heart disease, myocardial infarction, and in overall cardiovascular morbidity and mortality.

Various forms of supraventricular arrhythmias, such as premature atrial contractions, paroxysmal atrial tachycardia, and atrial fibrillation are routinely treated with and prevented by β-blockers and calcium-channel blockers. Some premature ventricular complexes may respond to β-blockers.

CONGESTIVE HEART FAILURE

Reduction in arterial pressure is perhaps quantitatively the most important treatment for hypertensive heart failure. Treatment of hypertension with a variety of different regimens in major antihypertensive trials showed a consistent reduction in the occurrence of congestive heart failure. (see Chapter I). However, more recently, the strategy for treating congestive cardiac failure in normotensive patients has incorporated the use of drugs developed to lower blood pressure in hypertension to achieve a reduction in afterload or the increased peripheral vascular resistance present in heart failure. The goal is to achieve balanced arterial and venous vasodilation while maintaining adequate perfusion of the brain, heart, and kidneys (Cohn et al, 1981).

The traditional initial therapy of congestive heart failure has included some form of diuresis, particularly if edema is present. Volume depletion by diuretics usually relieves acute cardiopulmonary congestion and edema but may result in compensatory peripheral and intrarenal vasoconstriction. These secondary changes to volume depletion are mediated, at least in part, by further activation of the renin-angiotensin-aldosterone system, with attendant increases in systemic vascular resistance, and contribute to the pathogenesis of congestive heart failure (Laragh, 1962).

110

Administration of an antihypertensive drug that causes vasodilation is rational in this patient population. Vasodilation reduces the elevated vascular resistance and increases cardiac output. Vasodilator therapy is rational in both the diuretic and nondiuretic-treated patient. The α_1-blockers, prazosin and terazosin, the direct vasodilator, hydralazine, and the ACE inhibitors, captopril and enalapril, have all been shown to be effective in congestive heart failure. Hydralazine, in patients more than 50 years of age or in individuals with impaired baroreflexes, may be used without a β-blocker (Veterans Administration Cooperative Study Group, 1981). In general, β-blockers and, to some extent, the calcium-channel blockers verapamil and diltiazem are not favored in this setting because of their negative inotropic effect on the heart (Lewis, 1983). A sizeable fraction of these patients will also have coronary artery disease and therefore may develop angina with increased heart rate. In one study, prazosin, hydralazine, and captopril were compared in patients with severe coronary artery disease and congestive heart failure (Rouleau et al, 1982). Captopril consistently lowered the heart rate-blood pressure product while reducing coronary blood flow and myocardial oxygen consumption. This resulted in a reduction in pulmonary capillary wedge pressure and increased cardiac output. Prazosin and hydralazine reduced the double product similarly but increased myocardial oxygen consumption in some. Although all three agents produced comparable hemodynamic changes, the greatest increases in cardiac output occurred with hydralazine, and the largest reductions in pulmonary capillary wedge pressure were observed in patients treated with prazosin. Captopril, however, produced the most consistent hemodynamic effects and reduction in myocardial oxygen consumption.

The ACE inhibitors, of which captopril has been the most widely studied, possess many of the ideal characteristics for treatment of hypertensive heart failure. These characteristics may be summarized as follows:

1. They are balanced arterial/venous vasodilators.

2. They do not produce sodium and water retention when used alone (in contrast to a direct vasodilator or α_1-blockers).

3. They do not induce reflex increase in heart rate when pressure is reduced (unlike direct vasodilators), even though these reflexes may be impaired in chronic heart failure.

4. They block aldosterone-mediated potassium loss (Nicholls et al, 1981), a major concern with concurrent diuretic and digitalis therapy.

5. They produce a consistently balanced reduction in myocardial oxygen consumption and arterial pressure in patients with coexisting coronary artery disease.

6. Captopril may improve renal blood flow acutely (Creager et al, 1981) and renal function chronically if blood pressure is not reduced excessively (Dzau et al, 1980); these changes are as good as or better than can be achieved with other agents (Pierpont and Cohn, 1981). In addition, differences between captopril and enalapril are emerging in terms of renal hemodynamic effects. For example, Packer et al (1986) have shown that in patients with heart failure, which may not be directly applicable to the hypertensive population, captopril produced greater benefit and less hypotension than enalapril.

THERAPY OF HYPERTENSION AND METABOLIC DISORDERS

Diabetes Mellitus It has been estimated that about 14% of hypertensive patients also have glucose intolerance or diabetes. Looked at from another vantage, diabetics have an increased incidence of hypertension when compared to nondiabetics (Barret-Connor et al, 1981). Moreover, a large fraction of conventional antihypertensive agents adversely affect glucose metabolism.

Thiazide diuretics have been known for more than 25 years to increase the risk of developing diabetes (Flamenbaum, 1983; Goldner et al, 1960), particularly in groups more likely to develop diabetes (Henningsen, 1984). Nonthiazides, such as the potassium-sparing diuretics (ie, spironolactone, triamterene, and amiloride) do not aggravate glucose tolerance in usual doses. On the other hand, the usefulness of these diuretics is limited by 1) their relatively low hypotensive potency at conventional doses, 2) their potential for inducing dangerous hyperkalemia in the setting of azotemia, a common consequence of diabetes and hypertension, and 3) their relative contraindication for use with converting-enzyme inhibitors, which also elevate serum potassium, particularly in patients with azotemic forms of renal disease. Maintaining or restoring to normal serum potassium may have particular importance in diabetics because there exists a strong correlation between reduction in total body potassium and defective insulin secretion (Roe et al, 1980). Thus, raising serum potassium with potassium-sparing diuretics and increased potassium salt ingestion reduces thiazide-related hyperglycemia (Helderman et al, 1983; Rapaport and Heard, 1964) and may correct the aberrations induced by thiazides so as not to need antidiabetes therapy (Grunfeld and Chappell, 1983). It is reasonable to propose, therefore, that the use of thiazides in diabetic patients should be accompanied with potassium-raising therapy such as oral potassium, potassium-sparing diuretics such as amiloride, triamterene, or spironolactone, or with a converting-enzyme inhibitor such as captopril or enalapril. Indapamide, a recently developed indolamine diuretic, may have less potential for inducing diabetes and possesses the potency of conventional thiazides (Perry, 1983).

β-Blockers may also increase plasma glucose levels and reduce serum insulin, being less likely with the cardioselective agents (Waal-Manning and Bolli, 1980). In a crossover trial, the nonselective β-blocker propranolol, in contrast to the cardioselective metoprolol, impaired glucose tolerance in noninsulin-dependent diabetes mellitus without changing concentrations of serum insulin, plasma glucagon, or free fatty acids nor altering peripheral insulin sensitivity at rest (Groop et al, 1982). β-Blockers also retard recovery from insulin-induced hypoglycemia (Abramson et al, 1966), and they block or blunt hypoglycemia-induced autonomic reflexes that are relied on to identify impending severe conditions. This latter action occurs more prominently with the nonselective β-blockers (Deacon et al, 1977).

The combined α-β-blocker, labetalol, does not appear to change glucose metabolism (Michelson et al, 1983), nor does the direct vasodilator hydralazine (Perry, 1983), with which β-blockers have been frequently combined. Clonidine also suppresses insulin release in diabetics and may aggravate diabetes (LeClercq-Meyers et al, 1980; Metz et al, 1983).

Calcium-channel blockers have also been associated with alterations in glucose metabolism. Both verapamil and nifedipine are associated with impaired insulin release (Lewis, 1983), and nifedipine has been shown to impair glucose tolerance (Charles et al, 1981). DeMarinis and Barbarino (1980) have shown that verapamil inhibits glucose-induced insulin secretion. The clinical implications of these findings remain to be clarified.

In contrast to these agents, Weinberger (1982) showed that the ACE inhibitor, captopril, did not affect insulin release or glucose metabolism. Captopril and enalapril are often used in combination with thiazide diuretics. This combination results in normalization of serum potassium (Sassano et al, 1984; Weinberger, 1983), leading to optimization of glucose and insulin metabolism. Significant new data related to the selective renal-sparing effect of converting-enzyme inhibitors is now available (see Chapter VIII). A number of major points of this section are summarized in Table II.

Uric Acid It has been appreciated for many years that thiazide diuretics raise serum uric acid in hypertension. For this reason, treatment with thiazides may precipitate acute gout or perpetuate chronic gout.

Table II.   Treatment of hypertension and diabetes mellitus.

Preferred therapy	Use with caution	Avoid
ACE inhibitor	Cardioselective β-blocker	Nonselective β-blocker
α_1-β-Blocker (labetalol)		
α_1-Blocker		
Potassium-sparing diuretic[a]	Calcium-channel blocker	
Thiazide diuretic or indapamide		
with: ACE inhibitor[a]		
OR		
potassium-sparing diuretic[a]		
OR		
potassium salt supplement[a]		

[a] Use with caution in azotemic patients.

Although pretreatment with allopurinol with or without colchicine may prevent thiazide-induced gout, it may be preferable to reduce blood pressure with another kind of agent. Nonthiazide diuretics may raise uric acid levels to a lesser degree due to hemoconcentration, as opposed to a direct effect on tubular secretion. Standard β-blockers may induce a slight rise in serum uric acid (Carr, 1984), whereas labetalol (Michelson et al, 1983), prazosin (Ram et al, 1981), and captopril (Weinberger, 1982, 1983) are generally neutral.

Lipid Metabolism   With the critical findings of the Lipid Research Clinics Program (1984), the roles of total cholesterol, low-density and high-density lipoproteins (LDL and HDL, respectively), along with free fatty acids (FFA) have become matters of pivotal interest in the prevention of cardiovascular disease. Recent important studies of changes in lipoproteins and lipid fractions by antihypertensive drugs have led to considerable debate over the strategy by which therapy is chosen (Freis, 1986; see Chapter II).

Thiazide diuretics raise LDL cholesterol and the LDL/HDL ratio (Ames, 1983a,b, 1984; Weidmann et al, 1983). However, indapamide and spironolactone appear to have minimal effects on lipoproteins (Weidmann et al, 1983). Interestingly, these latter authors also found that increases in LDL were prevented or reversed by concomitant β-blockade but not by reserpine, methyldopa, or clonidine. Wein-

Table III.   Treatment of hypertension and hypercholesterolemia.

Preferred therapy	Use with caution	Avoid
α_1-Blockers	Diuretics alone Spironolactone Indapamide	Thiazides alone

ACE inhibitor
  alone or with thiazide
	Thiazide with β-
	  blocker	

α-β-Blocker	β-Blocker	
Calcium-channel blocker Clonidine Guanabenz		

berger (1983) showed that captopril reversed or blunted the increase in cholesterol and LDL induced by thiazides.

β-Blockers have been shown to reduce HDL levels while increasing total triglycerides, very low density lipoproteins (VLDL) cholesterol, and FFA (Day et al, 1984). Labetalol, the combined β_1-blocker, appears to produce no change in serum lipids (Frishman et al, 1983). Pindolol, a β-blocker with partial agonist activity, raises HDL cholesterol without changing VLDL cholesterol (Pasotti et al, 1982).

α-Blockers produce variable effects on plasma lipids. Methyldopa reduces HDL (Ames and Hill, 1982), guanabenz may lower total cholesterol (Walker et al, 1981), while clonidine appears not to produce changes in serum lipids (Pagani et al, 1984). Calcium-channel blockers also appear to have a neutral effect on lipids and lipoproteins (Wada et al, 1982), as does the converting-enzyme inhibitor captopril (Weinberger, 1982). The peripheral α_1-blockers (ie, prazosin) all act to increase the HDL to total cholesterol ratio, lowering total cholesterol, LDL cholesterol, and raising HDL (Kokubu et al, 1982; Leren et al, 1980; Velasco et al, 1982). Moreover, these postsynaptic α-blockers partially correct the lipid disturbances induced by diuretics and β-blockers (Ferrier et al, 1986; Singleton and Taylor, 1983; Zanchetti, 1984). Altogether, the peripheral α-blockers appear to exert an overall positive effect on both hypertension and plasma lipids alone or in combination with other agents that may produce adverse changes. There is, however, no direct evidence, to date, that changing lipid concentrations with antihypertensive drugs alters the risk level for production of atherosclerosis. A summary of the main points of this discussion is found in Table III.

THERAPY OF HYPERTENSION AND PULMONARY DISEASE

Asthma   It has been estimated that at least 7% of hypertensive patients have asthma, and even more have cold-induced or exercise-induced bronchospasm.

There exist a number of important interactions between antihypertensive drugs and asthma and its treatment.

Diuretics appear to have no effect on airway reactivity (Light RW, et al, 1983) but may lead to salt depletion and dehydration and therefore aggravate asthma attacks. Diuretics, moreover, may produce hypokalemia, which may be worsened by treatment of asthma with epinephrine (Struthers et al, 1983), by β_2-agonists (Kung et al, 1984), or by corticosteroids. Since hypokalemia and hypomagnesemia induced by diuretic therapy may induce cardiac arrhythmias, these cations need to be replaced (Webster and Dyckner, 1981), particularly if cardiac disease exists or digitalis preparations are being used. Potent diuretics such as furosemide may increase theophylline concentrations and may require monitoring of serum theophylline levels (Conlon et al, 1981). Finally, diuretic-induced dehydration may lead to tenacious mucous that is difficult to clear.

β-Blockers, even cardioselective agents, increase airway resistance and thereby precipitate or aggravate asthma (Benson et al, 1978; Lawrence et al, 1982). In contrast, terazosin and presumably other α_1-blockers do not produce bronchospasm (Sperzel et al, 1986). Calcium-channel blockers act to blunt bronchoconstriction in response to certain stimuli (Corsis et al, 1983) and may, therefore, be beneficial. Although converting-enzyme inhibitors do not induce bronchospasm (Heel et al, 1980), there is a rare incidence of cough in some patients that has been reported to lead to bronchospasm (Salena, 1986; Semple and Herd, 1986). On the other hand, captopril blunts or blocks diuretic-induced hypokalemia (Weinberger, 1983) by its antialdosterone mechanism (Atlas et al, 1979), making this drug combination more potentially safe in the patient with asthma by producing neither bronchospasm or hypokalemia.

Chronic Obstructive Pulmonary Disease (COPD)   In patients with COPD, because thiazide diuretics may lead to sodium and chloride depletion, they contribute to hypokalemic alkalosis, frequently present in this population. This further elevates serum bicarbonate levels already increased through renal compensation of chronic respiratory acidosis. The superimposition of a metabolic alkalosis on a respiratory acidosis can lead to a marked alkalemia, which can, in turn, depress ventilatory drive (Hill, 1986). Thiazide diuretics also may lead to both potassium and magnesium deficiency and potentiate serious cardiac arrhythmias (Flink, 1981), digitalis toxicity (Webster and Dyckner, 1981), and weakening of respiratory muscles (Dhingra et al, 1984). In this patient population, ACE inhibitors are preferred therapy for coexistent hypertensives because they reduce blood pressure and block reactive aldosterone and thereby tend to normalize serum potassium (Weinberger, 1983).

Although both nonspecific and cardioselective β-blockers may increase airway resistance in COPD, in low doses, the cardioselective β-blocker atenolol (Benson et al, 1978) and the combined α-β-blocker labetalol (Anavekar et al, 1982; Light RW, et al, 1983) may be used successfully in some but not all mildly-to-moderately impaired patients.

Layton (1981) has shown that the α_1-blocker prazosin does not adversely affect pulmonary function in hypertensive patients with fixed airway disease. The calcium-channel blocker verapamil (Anavekar et al, 1982) and the converting-

115

Table IV.   Antihypertensive therapy in patients with pulmonary disease.

Condition	Preferred therapy	Avoid
Asthma	Calcium-channel blockers (nifedipine)	β-Blockers
	α_1-Blockers ACE inhibitors Diuretics[a]	
COPD[b]	α_1-Blockers ACE inhibitors Calcium-channel blockers	Nonselective β-blockers
	α-β Blockers[a] Cardioselective β-blockers[a] Diuretics[a]	

[a] Used cautiously; see text.
[b] COPD-chronic obstructive pulmonary disease

enzyme inhibitor captopril does not adversely affect ventilatory function in COPD and may increase vital capacity (Bertoli et al, 1985). A summary of the interaction of antihypertensive drugs and patients with pulmonary disease is found in Table IV.

TREATMENT OF HYPERTENSION WITH COEXISTING PERIPHERAL VASCULAR DISEASE

Obstructive vascular disease manifest either by reduced or absent pulses in the legs or by symptomatic claudication is common in older hypertensive patients. Although diuretic therapy has not been reported to worsen claudication, the increase in whole blood viscosity and reduced muscle flow may contribute to the frequent complaint of generalized or nocturnal leg cramps observed during diuretic therapy. On the other hand, the β-adrenergic blocker propranolol is commonly associated with worsening peripheral vascular disease (Forgoros, 1980). In one study by Ingram et al (1982), stopping selective or nonselective β-blockers with or without intrinsic sympathomimetic activity led to significant improvement in claudication distance and skin and muscle blood flow estimated by xenon-133 clearance improvement. Complications as severe as gangrene (Vale and Jeffreys, 1978) and skin necrosis (Gokal et al, 1979) have been described as complications of β-blockade. The reflex arterial vasospasm and the fall in FFA and glucose during exercise have been impugned in the pathophysiologic mechanisms of β-blockade-induced vasospasm (Goodfellow, 1980). Although β-blockers are commonly thought to worsen Raynaud's disease, one study showed that treatment with β-blockers was associated with an increased prevalence of cold extremities but not Raynaud's (Steiner et al, 1982). In a recent study, the α-β-blocker labetalol produced significantly fewer peripheral vascular side effects when compared to prior therapy with the standard β-blockers propranolol, nadolol, atenolol, pindolol, and metoprolol (Burris et al, 1986).

Selective α_1-blockers, such as prazosin, appear to be well tolerated in peripheral vascular disease and in patients with Raynaud's phenomenon or reflex cold sensitivity (Waldo, 1979). Similarly, converting-enzyme inhibitors may also improve peripheral circulation. In one case report, captopril produced both immediate and long-term benefit in a patient with Raynaud's phenomenon (Miyazaki et al, 1982). Captopril also reduced symptoms in some patients with hypertension and scleroderma (Whitman et al, 1982).

THERAPY OF HYPERTENSION AND COEXISTING RENAL DISEASE

The presence of azotemic renal disease commonly complicates the treatment of hypertension because many of the drugs used are cleared by the kidneys and there is a dose-related hemodynamic effect or toxicity. Azotemia, moreover, is a complication of hypertension usually resulting from nephrosclerosis. The ideal agent, therefore, should reduce arterial pressure but maintain renal blood flow and glomerular filtration and, in the long term, preserve nephrons and renal function. This discussion will address the immediate effects of antihypertensive drugs on renal function and blood flow and provide suggestions for therapy.

It is well established that thiazide diuretics may induce significant volume contraction causing azotemia to develop or worsen while increasing uric acid. This may be limited to some extent by prevention of excessive volume depletion, as can occur when diuretic therapy is combined with a very low sodium intake. Because salt and water retention accompany most forms of renal disease, diuretics are often effective antihypertensive agents, particularly in more advanced renal insufficiency. Thiazide diuretics are adequate when azotemia is mild, but the loop diuretics, furosemide, ethacrynic acid, bumetanide, and metazolone, and indapamide are more effective when renal function has declined. In general, the potassium-conserving agents spironolactone, triamterene, amiloride, and their combinations with thiazide diuretics should be avoided with advancing renal insufficiency, which is associated with impaired potassium excretion.

Diuretics, in general, decrease glomerular filtration rate and renal blood flow (Roos et al, 1981) in hypertensive patients. Renal cortical blood flow is already reduced in nonazotemic hypertension (Hollenberg et al, 1978, 1981) but can be normalized by intravenous saline loading (deLeeuw and Birkenhager, 1983). Since the reduction in renal blood flow reflects, in part, renal cortical vasoconstriction, vigorous diuresis alone may lead to worsening azotemia by markedly stimulating the renin-angiotensin-aldosterone system, which further diminishes cortical blood flow. Thus, in patients with renal disease, it is rational to use a diuretic without producing excessive volume depletion and to combine it with a second drug that preserves or increases renal blood flow and function. This is particularly needed if the second drug produces sodium retention by itself. Drugs that may lead to sodium and water retention are shown in Table V.

117

Table V.   Antihypertensive drug effects on sodium retention.

Natriuresis-diuresis	Neutral	Sodium/water retention
Diuretics		Direct vasodilators[a]
	β-Blockers	
	ACE inhibitors	
	α-Blockers	
	Calcium-channel blockers[b]	

[a] Rarely used alone; generally combined with diuretic and β-blocker.
[b] May cause edema in lower extremities but not by causing renal sodium and water retention.

Individual β-blockers produce variable effects on renal function, variations that are independent of their cardioselectivity or partial agonist activity. In usual antihypertensive doses, however, β-blockers rarely cause renal function to deteriorate clinically. Propranolol reduces renal blood flow (Bauer and Brooks, 1979). In contrast, nadolol either does not change or relatively increases renal blood flow (O'Malley et al, 1983). Other β-blockers, including atenolol (Waal-Manning and Bolli, 1980), pindolol (Kostis and DeFelice, 1983), timolol (Malini et al, 1983), and labetalol (O'Malley et al, 1983), appear to exert little change on renal blood flow or function.

The central α-agonists clonidine and methyldopa do not reduce renal blood flow (Morin et al, 1964; Onesti, 1978). However, the peripheral α_1-blockers prazosin and trimazosin either do not change or may improve glomerular filtration and renal blood flow in hypertensive patients with and without azotemia (Chrysant et al, 1980; O'Connor et al, 1978; Preston et al, 1979).

The ACE inhibitors have also been shown to maintain or increase renal blood flow (Bauer, 1984; Johnston, 1984). However, if the hypertension is caused by severe bilateral renal artery stenoses or stenosis of a solitary kidney's renal artery, a deterioration of renal function or even frank renal failure that is usually reversible can occur in the setting of sodium-volume depletion (Hricik et al, 1983).

Calcium-channel blockers may produce deleterious intrarenal hemodynamic alterations in patients with impaired renal function. Nifedipine produced acute reversible renal deterioration in patients with hypertension and mild azotemia (Diamond et al, 1984). This has been attributed, in part, to the drug's ability to block angiotensin II stimulation of prostaglandin E_2 synthesis, believed to be critically protective of renal function (Ausiello and Zusman, 1984; Blum et al, 1981).

Table VI. **Miscellaneous chronic medical conditions and antihypertensive drugs.**

Condition	Drugs that may help	Drugs that may worsen
Osteoporosis	Thiazide diuretics	
Calcium stone disease	Thiazide diuretics	
Chronic rhinitis or sinusitis	–	Central α-agonists α_1-Blockers
Insomnia	Central α-agonists	Lipid-soluble β-blockers
Male sexual dysfunction	–	Spironolactone Thiazide diuretics β-Blockers Central α-agonists
Migraine headaches	Lipid-soluble β-blockers Central α-agonists	Hydralazine
Functional diarrhea	Verapamil Diltiazem Central α-agonists	β-blockers (vagomimetic)
Esophageal spasm/dysmotility	Nifedipine	–
Baldness	Minoxidil	β-Blockers
Sicca syndrome	–	α-Blockers

119

TREATMENT OF HYPERTENSION AND OTHER MISCELLANEOUS MEDICAL CONDITIONS

Table VI summarizes a group of selected chronic medical conditions and the interaction with antihypertensive drugs.

CONCLUSIONS

This chapter has emphasized the usefulness of considering the whole patient—his or her coexisting medical conditions and personal needs—as a basis for selecting initial therapy. This process is somewhat different from the impersonal algorithm set forth by the Joint National Committee (1984) by not being restricted in the selection of any first or second agent.

The issues of cost and convenience have not been fully discussed. When compared to the other expenses of daily living—or even the costs, inconvenience, risks, or complications from poorly conceived therapy—there are relatively few instances where the price of a drug should be a deterrent to proper therapy. Convenience is another important consideration for a majority of patients, with once-daily regimens being the most suitable. Many β-blockers, diuretics, one calcium-channel blocker (sustained-release verapamil), and ACE inhibitors are effective when administered once daily. It is likely that a number of currently investigational long-acting calcium-channel blockers, combined α-β-blockers, and peripheral α-blockers will also be available in the near future.

For the majority of patients with mild essential hypertension without significant other medical problems, the most neutral class of antihypertensive drugs is the ACE inhibitors, followed by the α-β-blockers, peripheral α-blockers, and the calcium-channel blockers. By neutral, it is meant absence of either symptomatic side effects or chemical aberrations or effects other than lowering arterial pressure. In addition, there is a growing body of evidence to suggest that some of these drugs may have other special beneficial effects beyond the reduction of blood pressure per se in conserving renal function, improving blood lipid profiles, arresting or reducing cardiac hypertrophy, and in improving the quality of life. Thus, the selection of antihypertensive therapy requires a careful medical and personal appraisal as a basis for a rational individualized strategy. This approach does not require sophisticated hemodynamic or hormonal testing for the majority of patients but rather for the few who have severe or treatment-resistant hypertension or other clues suggestive of a secondary form of hypertension.

Chapter VII

Diabetes and Hypertension: Considerations for Therapy

Leopoldo Raij, MD, and Jonathan P. Tolins, MD

INTRODUCTION

Patients with Type I or insulin-dependent diabetes mellitus (IDDM) or Type II diabetes mellitus (DM), noninsulin dependent, are at increased risk for the development of arterial hypertension. When hypertension is superimposed on DM, the risk for the morbid consequences of cerebrovascular and coronary atherosclerosis, as well as the specific microvascular complications of DM, retinopathy, and nephropathy, are increased. Thus, control of blood pressure assumes utmost importance in the diabetic, and the physician caring for these patients will frequently be required to make decisions regarding antihypertensive therapy. Therapeutic decisions must be guided not only by efficacy in lowering blood pressure but by effects on carbohydrate metabolism, specific diabetic symptoms (eg, orthostatic hypotension), and possibly by hemodynamic responses in the microvasculature of the organs at risk.

THE RELATIONSHIP BETWEEN DIABETES AND HYPERTENSION

Prevalence of Hypertension in the Diabetic Patient Although the association of hypertension and DM is clinically apparent, defining the extent of the problem epidemiologically has proved difficult. Possible complicating factors include age, obesity, presence of renal disease, and the use of specialty clinic patients (Fuller, 1985a).

Large-scale surveys of young patients with IDDM suggest an increased incidence of hypertension (Christlieb et al, 1981; Moss, 1962). In a long-term follow-up study of 1072 patients with IDDM (White, 1956), hypertension eventually developed in 53% of patients, and its onset was closely paralleled by the development of retinopathy and nephropathy. Young diabetics with completely normal renal function often have normal blood pressure (Feldt-Rasmussen et al, 1985), while even "incipient" diabetic nephropathy, defined by the presence of microalbuminuria (20 μg/min to 70 μg/min of urinary albumin excretion), is associated with increased blood pressure (Table I; Mogensen, 1987). In patients

Table I. **Stages of diabetic nephropathy (from Mogensen, 1987, with permission).**

Stage	Designation	Main characteristics	Main structural changes
Stage I	Hyperfunction and hypertrophy stage[b]	Large kidneys and glomerular hyperfiltration	Glomerular hypertrophy normal base-ment membrane and mesangium
Stage II			
In short-term diabetes (2–15 years)	"Silent" stage with normal UAE but structural lesion present	Normal UAE	Increasing membrane (bm) thickness and mesangial expansion
In long-term diabetes			No or few studies
Stage III			
Early			
	Incipient DN[a]	Persistently elevated UAE	Severity probably inbetween II and IV
Late			
Stage IV			
Early		Clinical proteinuria or UAE >200 μg/min <200 μg/min	Increasing rate of glomerular closure
Intermediate	Overt DN		Hypertrophy of remaining glomeruli (as in III)
Advanced			
Stage V	Uremia	End-stage renal failure	Generalized glomerular closure

[a] GFR — glomerular filtration rate; UAE — urinary albumin excretion; DN — diabetic nephropathy.
[b] Changes present probably in all stages when control imperfect.
[c] Marker of future nephropathy (if GFR > 150 ml/min).

GFR[a] (ml/ min)	Albumin excretion (UAE)[a]	Blood pressure	Suggested main pathophysio- logic change
≈150	May be increased	N (may fall initially during insulin treatment	Glomerular volume expansion and increased intraglomerular pressure
With or without hyperfiltration[c]	N (often increased in stress situations	N	Changes as indicated above but quite variable (dependent on metabolic control?)
With or without hyperfiltration[c]	N (often increased in stress situations	N or slightly elevated	In addition, increased synthesis of bm and bm-like-material
≈160	20–70 μg/min	Often elevated compared to healthy subjects; also blood pressure elevated during exercise	Glomerular closure probably starts in this stage
≈130	70–200		
≈130– 70	>200 μg/min	Often frank hypertension	High rate of glomerular closure and advancing mesangial
≈70–30		Hypertension almost ubiquitous	
≈30–10		Hypertension almost ubiquitous	Hyperfiltration in remaining glomeruli (deleterious)
0–10	Decreasing	High but controlled by dialysis treatment	Advanced lesions and glomerular closure

123

with IDDM and established nephropathy, hypertension is ubiquitous (Parving et al, 1981). Thus, in IDDM, the development of hypertension is closely linked to the onset of renal injury, and its prevalence should be expected to reflect the frequency of diabetic nephropathy in this population.

In patients with Type II, usually adult-onset DM (AODM), the prevalence of hypertension is 40% to 53% in the clinic setting (Turner, 1985). This increased prevalence of hypertension in AODM has also been found in population studies when such confounding factors as age, sex, and obesity are taken into account (Pell and D'Alanza, 1967). As discussed below, the factors responsible for the increased frequency of elevated blood pressure in AODM are uncertain and may reflect specific abnormalities of the diabetic milieu (eg, hyperinsulinemia and subsequent sodium retention) or an increased incidence of essential hypertension in this population.

Hypertension as a Risk Factor in the Diabetic Patient   Diabetic patients have a clear propensity for the development of diffuse atherosclerotic vascular disease, with frequently devastating consequences. Several prospective studies have shown that hypertension is an important risk factor for diabetic macrovascular disease (Fuller, 1985b). In the Whitehall study of male civil servants (Fuller et al, 1983), a ten-year follow-up revealed a significant upward trend in coronary heart disease (CHD) mortality in diabetics with increasing systolic blood pressure. Analysis showed that age and systolic blood pressure were the major contributors to the increased risk of CHD death in subjects with glucose intolerance and with overt DM (Figure 1). In a study of Finnish men (Aromaa et al, 1984), hypertensive diabetics had a relative risk of CHD mortality of 4.69 in comparison to normotensive nondiabetics. Other studies have also shown that hypertension in the diabetic patient is clearly associated with increased morbidity and mortality from cerebrovascular and peripheral vascular disease (Duncan and Faris, 1986; Fuller et al, 1983; Roehmoldt et al, 1983).

The weight of evidence also suggests that hypertension increases the incidence and rate of progression of the microvascular complications specific to DM: retinopathy and nephropathy. In a six-year follow-up of Pima Indians, the incidence of retinal exudates was doubled in hypertensive, as compared to normotensive, diabetics (Knowler et al, 1980), a finding noted in other populations as well (Lombrail et al, 1983).

Elevated blood pressure is present even in the earliest detectable stages of diabetic nephropathy (Mogensen, 1987; Parving et al, 1983a). Two studies have suggested that antihypertensive therapy can slow the rate of progression of established diabetic nephropathy (Mogensen, 1983; Parving et al, 1983b). Thus, it is clear that elevated arterial blood pressure is intimately related to the development and progression of renal impairment in patients with DM.

The evidence therefore suggests that control of hypertension is of major importance in the diabetic patient. If instituted early in the course of the disease, adequate treatment could potentially protect the patients from the adverse consequences of diffuse atherosclerosis and delay the onset and progression of specific diabetic microvascular disease.

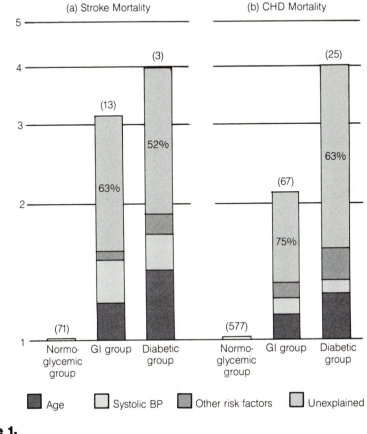

Figure 1.
Relative risks (odds-ratios) of (a) stroke death and (b) coronary
heart disease death explained by risk factors (age-standardized) for
(1) the glucose intolerance group and (2) the diabetic group
compared to the normoglycemic group. Figures at top of columns
are numbers of deaths. Only subjects with complete information
are included (from Fuller et al, 1983, with permission).

125

The Pathogenesis of Hypertension in Diabetes In considering the underlying mechanisms leading to hypertension in diabetic patients, the two types of disease must be considered separately. In patients with IDDM, hypertension is intimately related to the development of diabetic nephropathy. It is likely that systemic blood pressure rises only when structural changes in the glomerulus have become established (Mogensen, 1987). Elevated blood pressure was noted at initial evaluation in patients with IDDM who subsequently developed overt nephropathy but not in those patients in whom renal function remained normal (Mogensen and Christensen, 1984). Furthermore, recent studies (Krolewski et al, 1987) have shown that genetic predisposition to hypertension is a major determinant of diabetic nephropathy. In patients with IDDM and established nephropathy, the rate of decline in renal function is proportional to the level of diastolic blood pressure (Mogensen, 1976a,b). In these patients, elevated blood pressure is both a reflection of underlying renal disease and a major factor causing progression of nephropathy.

The cause of hypertension in patients with AODM is less clear. These patients often have peripheral insulin resistance and hyperinsulinemia. It has been shown (De Fronzo, 1981) that increased insulin levels within the physiologic range stimulate renal sodium retention. Hence, it was postulated that sodium retention may be a factor in the development of hypertension in these patients. Results of studies determining total body or exchangeable sodium in diabetics with hypertension have been variable but generally show a significant increase of about 10% (Chatel et al, 1977; Weidmann et al, 1985). Patients with diabetes and hypertension have increased influx of sodium into red blood cells when compared to normotensive diabetics and controls (Chimori et al, 1986), suggesting intracellular accumulation of sodium. Thus, abnormalities in sodium balance and distribution are associated with DM and may explain, at least in part, the cardiovascular hyperreactivity of diabetic patients, such as increased pressor response to angiotensin II and norepinephrine (Christlieb et al, 1976a; Weidmann et al, 1985). Others have emphasized the importance of decreased activity of the renal kallikrein-kinin system in the pathogenesis of diabetic hypertension (Mitas et al, 1978; Olshan et al, 1982).

A number of studies have found abnormalities of various levels of the renin-angiotensin system in patients with DM and hypertension. In general, normal plasma renin activity (PRA) has been found in diabetics with hypertension who have no evidence of renal disease while diabetics with nephropathy have decreased PRA (Christlieb et al, 1976b). Possible explanations for the low PRA include volume expansion due to sodium/fluid retention, hyaline destruction of the cells of the juxtaglomerular apparatus as part of the renal parenchymal disease, decreased renin release due to decreased circulating levels of catecholamines and autonomic neuropathy, and decreased conversion of prorenin to active renin (Christlieb, 1976; DeLeive et al, 1976). Given the increased total body exchangeable sodium in diabetics with hypertension, it is possible that the observed normal, or even low, levels of renin activity are inappropriately high and play a role in the maintenance of high blood pressure. However, in diabetic nephropathy, as in other chronic renal parenchymal diseases, a correlation between circulating renin levels and blood pressure has not been consistently found (Beretta-Piccoli et al, 1976). Moreover, recent studies have emphasized the importance of the vascular renin-angiotensin pathway in the pathogenesis of hypertension, the activity of which may not be reflected by the PRA (Dzau, 1986). Thus, the importance of abnormalities in the renin-angiotensin system in hypertension associated with DM remains unclear.

DIABETIC NEPHROPATHY: ROLE OF HEMODYNAMIC AND METABOLIC FACTORS

Diabetic nephropathy, defined as the appearance of proteinuria, elevated arterial blood pressure, and diminished glomerular filtration rate, will develop in as many as 45% of patients with IDDM (Andersen et al, 1983). In patients with the onset of diabetes at an early age, renal disease is an important contributor to mortality, accounting for up to 31% of all deaths (Deckert et al, 1978). Renal disease also complicates DM developing in adults and contributes significantly to morbidity and mortality in this group (Knowles, 1974). In both types of DM, the appearance of clinically detectable proteinuria (more than 200 μg/min of urinary albumin excretion) signals the onset and relentless progression of diabetic nephropathy, which is typically followed by deterioration of renal function culminating in end-stage renal disease (Table I). The pathogenesis of diabetic nephropathy has been recently reviewed in detail elsewhere (Hostetter, 1986). For the purposes of this discussion, diabetic nephropathy can be seen to be the result of metabolic abnormalities inherent to diabetes (eg, hyperglycemia) and hemodynamic abnormalities of the renal microcirculation that result in progressive structural and functional glomerular abnormalities.

Strict control of blood glucose prevents the appearance of diabetic microangiopathy in experimental animals (Mauer et al, 1975), but the effect of this therapeutic maneuver in patients with diabetes is less clear. When diabetic nephropathy is clearly established (ie, clinically detectable proteinuria), even prolonged strict metabolic control achieved with continuous insulin infusion techniques does not affect the rate of deterioration of renal function in patients with IDDM (Viberti et al, 1983). However, when strict metabolic control is imposed on patients with early or incipient nephropathy, as defined by the presence of microalbuminuria, 20 μg/min to 70 μg/min of urinary albumin excretion (Mogensen, 1987), progression to overt nephropathy can be arrested, at least temporarily (Feldt-Rasmussen et al, 1986). Thus, metabolic factors may be critical in the early stages of diabetic nephropathy, but by the time glomerular function has started to fail, the process leading to eventual renal failure is self-perpetuating and not significantly affected even by strict metabolic control.

In experimental models of diabetes, glomerular hyperfiltration associated with increased intraglomerular pressures and flows appears responsible for the development and progression of diabetic nephropathy (Hostetter et al, 1982). Experimental maneuvers known to increase intraglomerular pressure, such as contralateral uninephrectomy (Steffes et al, 1978) or high protein feeding (Zatz et al, 1985), have been shown to accelerate renal injury in experimental diabetic nephropathy. In fact, in experimental diabetes, glomerular flows and pressures are increased even when systemic blood pressure is normal. This is due to an imbalance in the interaction between those hemodynamic determinants that control the glomerular microcirculation, namely, afferent and efferent vascular resistances, and the glomerular capillary ultrafiltration coefficient. Moreover, in diabetes, a relative deficiency in preglomerular resistances may permit the occurrence of disproportionate rises in glomerular pressures even when elevations in systemic hypertension are small. This will explain the exquisite sensitivity of

127

the diabetic kidney to hypertension (Figure 2; Mauer et al, 1978; Mogensen, 1976b). Understanding of these renal hemodynamic changes not only has pathophysiologic connotations but also therapeutic implications. Experimentally, converting-enzyme inhibitors have consistently been shown to effectively lower systemic as well as glomerular hypertension and concomitantly reduce the progression of glomerular injury in chronic renal failure and in diabetes (Anderson et al, 1986; Raij, 1986; Raij et al, 1985; Zatz et al, 1986). Converting enzyme inhibition decreases glomerular efferent arteriole constriction and increases the ultrafiltration coefficient. These effects result in maintenance of glomerular blood flow and glomerular filtration rate with concomitant fall in intraglomerular pressure (Anderson et al, 1986). Whether the suggested beneficial effects of converting-enzyme inhibition are exclusively due to changes in intraglomerular hemodynamic factors or to an added effect of these drugs upon intraglomerular structures, particularly the mesangium, is at present unknown (Raij and Keane, 1985).

Similar hemodynamic alterations to those observed in animals have been postulated to occur in patients with DM (Mogensen, 1976b). In a long-term follow-up study of patients with IDDM who had no evidence of nephropathy at initial evaluation, those patients who showed evidence of progression to clinical diabetic nephropathy had an elevated glomerular filtration rate (GFR) early in their course (Mogensen and Christensen, 1984). In patients who subsequently developed overt nephropathy, arterial blood pressure was elevated initially and increased significantly during the follow-up period. The investigators concluded that glomerular hyperfiltration and elevated glomerular pressures likely were involved in the pathogenesis of human diabetic nephropathy. Other studies demonstrated that when DM is complicated by hypertension, the rate of decline of renal function is accelerated (Mogensen, 1976a; Parving et al, 1983b) and that when blood pressure is controlled, progression of nephropathy can be slowed or arrested (Mogensen, 1983; Parving et al, 1983b).

From the above discussion, it is apparent that if the adverse consequences of diabetic nephropathy are to be avoided, the clinician must aggressively control arterial blood pressure from a very early stage in the disease process; agents that lower both systemic and glomerular capillary pressure would be particularly advantageous. It is also apparent that, especially in the early stages of the disease, this must be done without adversely affecting metabolic control. Thus, the treatment of hypertension in the diabetic patient becomes both critically important and problematic.

THERAPY OF HYPERTENSION IN DIABETES MELLITUS

Nondrug Therapy Although the patient with DM and hypertension will typically require pharmacologic antihypertensive therapy, there are nonpharmacologic measures that are clearly useful in improving blood pressure response to drug treatment. In patients with AODM, hypertension is frequently associated with obesity (Modan et al, 1985). Weight loss can be beneficial in blood pressure control in obese, noninsulin-dependent diabetics (Heyden, 1978). Several studies have suggested that increased physical activity may be beneficial in the control

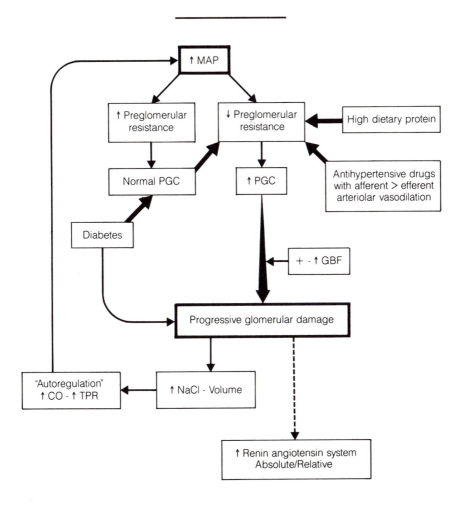

Figure 2.
Scheme of the relationship between hypertension and glomerular injury in diabetic nephropathy. MAP = mean arterial pressure; PGC = glomerular capillary pressure; GBF = glomerular blood flow; CO = cardiac output; TPR = total peripheral resistance. (Figure 2 modified from "Role of Hypertension in Progressive Glomerular Injury in Glomerulonephritis". *Hypertension* **(suppl 1) Volume 8, No. 4, l30-l33, April 1986). (From Raij, 1986, with permission.)**

of hypertension associated with AODM (Siscovick et al, 1985). One study (Pacy et al, 1984) compared the effects of a high fiber, low fat, low sodium diet with thiazide diuretic therapy in diabetic patients with mild hypertension. Both groups had a similar decrease in blood pressure; however, the dietary group showed improvement in glycemic control and lipid profiles while these parameters tended to worsen in thiazide-treated patients. Modest salt restriction, to 3g to 5g of salt a day, can be effective in lowering blood pressure and in enhancing the action of diuretic and other antihypertensive drugs (Parijs et al, 1973; Tobian, 1978). However, care must be taken in patients with renal parenchymal disease to adjust the salt intake to the ability of the impaired kidney to maintain sodium balance and so avoid the extremes of dehydration and sodium/volume overload. Thus, it seems prudent to advise patients to achieve ideal weight by a combination of diet and exercise and to adhere to a diet modestly restricted in salt. While these measures may not normalize blood pressure in this patient population, they will enhance the efficacy and/or minimize the need for drug therapy.

Selection of Antihypertensive Drug Therapy The ultimate goal of antihypertensive drug therapy in the hypertensive diabetic is to avoid or arrest the morbid consequences of generalized macrovascular disease and diabetic microvascular disease (retinopathy and nephropathy). Thus, the ideal drug should be efficacious in lowering blood pressure, devoid of adverse effects on the metabolic control of diabetes, and perhaps have the added effect of lowering intraglomerular capillary pressure in addition to systemic blood pressure.

Thiazide Diuretics As noted above, hypertension in the diabetic is associated with normal to low PRA, in part due to increased exchangeable sodium and volume expansion. Therefore, diuretics would seem to be logical choices for antihypertensive therapy and indeed are effective in lowering blood pressure. Unfortunately, these drugs have been associated with adverse metabolic effects that may limit their use in some patients. In 1960, a study first drew attention (Goldner et al, 1960) to the hyperglycemic effect of thiazide diuretics. Twenty diabetic and 20 nondiabetic patients were given relatively high doses of thiazide diuretics. While none of the nondiabetic patients developed hyperglycemia or glycosuria, 6 of the 20 diabetics developed worsening hyperglycemia within three to five days of starting the drug. Another study (Dornhorst et al, 1985) noted a 31% increase in fasting blood sugar and a 6% increase in glycosated hemoglobin in patients with AODM and hypertension who were treated with hydrochlorothiazide. Others (Struthers et al, 1985) have since confirmed that the deterioration in glucose tolerance after thiazide diuretics appears to be greater in those patients who already have impaired glucose tolerance and that this is usually an early effect. A similar deterioration in glucose tolerance has been noted with the structurally related diuretic furosemide (Touvonen and Mustala, 1966).

The mechanism of thiazide-induced glucose intolerance is unclear. It seems likely that hypokalemia is at least contributory (Struthers et at, 1985) because it can be reversed with potassium supplementation (Rapaport and Heard, 1964). Recent studies (Rowe et al, 1980) using the glucose clamp technique noted decreased insulin response to a glucose load in normal subjects who were potassium depleted. In this study, tissue sensitivity to insulin was unchanged. Thus, the most likely explanation for thiazide-induced glucose intolerance is decreased pancreatic insulin release due to hypokalemia. This effect is unlikely to affect glycemic control in insulin-dependent patients with little or no pancreatic reserve. Thiazide diuretics also adversely affect serum cholesterol and triglyceride levels, as well as uric acid levels (Ames, 1984; Schoenfeld and Goldberger, 1964), all known risk factors for CHD. In the Multiple Risk Factor Intervention Trial [MRFIT] (MRFIT Research Group, 1982), thiazide treatment of hypertension may have been responsible for the increased total and CHD mortality seen in men with initial abnormal electrocardiograms, possibly due to hypokalemia and the other adverse metabolic effects noted above. Thus, in diabetic patients, thiazide diuretics may have unwanted effects that at times may outweigh their benefits.

Adrenergic Receptor Antagonists   Although the β-adrenergic receptor blocking agents are effective antihypertensive agents in patients with DM (Mogensen, 1983; Parving et al, 1983b), there are theoretical disadvantages to the use of these drugs. In patients on insulin therapy, the signs and symptoms of insulin-induced hypoglycemia are mediated by sympathoadrenal activity. Therefore, β-blockers may diminish awareness of incipient hypoglycemia and potentially lead to increased incidence of severe hypoglycemic episodes. There are, however, numerous clinical studies demonstrating that these drugs can be used safely and effectively in diabetic patients on insulin. One study (Blohm et al, 1981) compared metoprolol, a β_1-selective blocker, to placebo in five insulin-dependent diabetics with mild hypertension, all of whom were prone to hypoglycemic attacks. During treatment with the β-blocker, no increase in the number of severe hypoglycemic episodes was observed, although one patient noted slight masking of symptoms during hypoglycemia. In a study of patients with AODM followed for up to eight months, no increased frequency of severe hypoglycemic episodes was found in patients on β-blockers compared to controls (Barnett et al, 1980).

In the untreated diabetic, hypoglycemia induces catecholamine release with β_2-receptor-mediated vasodilation and mild decreases in diastolic blood pressure. Nonselective β-blockade can lead to unopposed α-receptor stimulation, with subsequent vasoconstriction and a marked pressor response (Barnett et al, 1980). This potentially adverse effect is not seen with β_1-selective blockers (Lloyd-Mostyn and Oram, 1975; Ostman et al, 1982). Thus, evidence suggests that β-adrenergic receptor blockers can be used safely and effectively in hypertensive diabetics; however, it seems prudent to use β-selective blockers.

131

α_2-adrenergic receptors are involved in the regulation of pancreatic insulin release (Struthers et al, 1985), thus, specific α_1-receptor antagonists such as prazosin would not be expected to adversely affect glucose tolerance. The antihypertensive response and affect on glucose tolerance of prazosin therapy in nondiabetic as well as diabetic hypertensive patients have been studied (Shionoiri et al, 1986). Long-term therapy resulted in a significant antihypertensive response and no deterioration in glucose tolerance in either group of patients. It was concluded that prazosin could be used safely and effectively in hypertensive diabetics.

Clonidine, a centrally acting α-agonist, was effective in blood pressure control in a group of patients with AODM and mild hypertension but significantly impaired the response to acute glucose challenge. However, the clinical significance of this effect on long-term diabetic control was negligible (Guthrie et al, 1983).

Calcium-channel Blockers   Insulin secretion is dependent on calcium influx into the pancreatic islet cell, hence, calcium-channel blockers might be expected to interfere with insulin secretion. However, Trost et al (1985) noted no adverse effect on glucose tolerance or lipid metabolism in hypertensive diabetic patients given a calcium antagonist at a dose that normalized blood pressure. This potential adverse effect would be less relevant in insulin-treated patients. Although enough experience is not available (Romero et al, 1987), this class of drugs may indeed be useful in the management of hypertension in diabetics, either singly or most likely complementing other antihypertensive agents, such as converting-enzyme inhibitors and/or diuretics.

Converting-enzyme Inhibitors   As noted above, diabetic hypertension is in general characterized by low PRA. However, PRA may still be inappropriately high for the increased total body sodium content of these patients (Chatel et al, 1977; Weidmann et al, 1985). It should be kept in mind that PRA may not reflect the state of activity of the intrarenal or vascular renin-angiotensin systems. The local actions of this system may in fact be more relevant than plasma levels to 1) the maintenance of elevated blood pressure (Dzau, 1986) and/or 2) the relationship between angiotensin II and glomerular injury (Keane and Raij, 1985; Raij and Keane, 1985). In addition, some studies have also suggested an increased sensitivity to the pressor effects of angiotensin II in diabetic patients with hypertension (Christlieb et al, 1976a). Thus, it can be expected that angiotensin converting enzyme inhibitors would be effective drugs in these patients. Furthermore, it is suggested that this class of agents may offer particular advantages in the prevention of onset and progression of diabetic nephropathy due to its specific reduction of intraglomerular capillary pressure (Anderson et al, 1986; Zatz et al, 1986).

Of the two converting-enzyme inhibitors currently available to the clinician, captopril and enalapril, the majority of the experience to date has been with captopril.

In a recent study, 20 hypertensive diabetic patients, both insulin-dependent and noninsulin-dependent, were treated with captopril for 12 weeks (D'Angelo et al, 1986). Sixteen patients responded with normalization of blood pressure with captopril alone, whereas the remaining four patients required the addition of a thiazide diuretic. No deterioration in the metabolic control of diabetes was noted. In another study (Dominguez et al, 1986), the effects of captopril in 16 hypertensive patients with AODM were studied. Captopril was effective as monotherapy in 53% of patients; the remaining patients responded after addition of a thiazide diuretic. Interestingly, in this study, significant improvement in the glucose response to an oral glucose tolerance test with a trend toward improved insulin response was noted; glycosylated hemoglobin levels improved during captopril therapy. Moreover, in hypertensive patients, captopril was found to ameliorate the adverse metabolic effects of thiazide diuretics when given in combination with these agents (Weinberger, 1985). One study (Ferriere et al, 1985) reported three cases of unexplained hypoglycemia in diabetic patients when captopril was added to their usual insulin dose. These investigators subsequently studied diabetic and nondiabetic patients with the glucose clamp technique before and after ten days of treatment with captopril and suggested that captopril enhanced insulin sensitivity. These findings were confirmed in another study (Rett et al, 1986) in which increased peripheral insulin sensitivity was found in patients with AODM after a single 25 mg dose of captopril. In aggregate, these studies suggest that captopril is effective in the treatment of hypertension in diabetic patients and may actually improve glucose tolerance via enhancement of peripheral insulin sensitivity.

The renal effects of converting-enzyme inhibition are an important consideration in the diabetic population. In diabetic rats, inhibition of angiotensin-converting enzymes with enalapril decreased glomerular capillary pressure and proteinuria (Zatz et al, 1986). Clinically, the renal effects of captopril were studied in 15 patients with established diabetic nephropathy and hypertension (Bjork et al, 1986). After nine days of therapy, these patients demonstrated no change in GFR but had a significant increase in renal plasma flow, implying a decrease in filtration fraction and hence suggesting a decrease in glomerular capillary hydraulic pressure. After two years of follow-up, the rate of deterioration of GFR in the captopril-treated diabetics had decreased from a loss of 10.3 ml/min/yr to only 2.4 ml/min/yr. Thus, converting-enzyme inhibition had a beneficial effect on the progression of diabetic nephropathy most likely due, as in the diabetic rats, to a beneficial effect on renal hemodynamic and/or glomerular structures (Anderson et al, 1986; Keane and Raij, 1985; Raij and Keane, 1985; Raij et al, 1985; Zatz et al, 1986). Captopril has also been studied in patients with IDDM and early nephropathy (Hommel et al, 1986). After 12 weeks of therapy, blood pressure and albuminuria had significantly decreased, and again, no significant change in GFR was noted. Even in advanced diabetic nephropathy with azotemia, captopril has been reported to decrease proteinuria (Taguma et al, 1985). The effect of this converting-enzyme inhibitor upon the glomerular microcirculation likely explains its renal protective effect beyond the benefit due to lowering systemic blood pressure. Indeed, preliminary studies (Ruilope et al, 1987) have shown that in patients with chronic renal failure in whom hypertension was controlled with a combination of a β-blocker vasodilator and a diuretic, the rate of decline in renal function was greatly diminished after switching to captopril. In summary, it appears that converting-enzyme inhibition can be used in diabetics at any stage of nephropathy, and available information is intriguing and persuasive. Their potential in arresting and/or reducing the progression of diabetic nephropathy, their efficacy in control of blood pressure, and their lack of adverse effects on the metabolic control of diabetes make converting-enzyme inhibitors an appealing choice in the diabetic patient with hypertension. At present, two large clinical trials are underway to assess the impact of converting-enzyme inhibition on the natural history of diabetic nephropathy. These results will be sought with interest.

133

CONCLUSIONS

It is apparent that if the morbid consequences of macrovascular and microvascular disease are to be minimized in the diabetic patient, then control of arterial hypertension must be a major goal from the earliest stages of the disease process. Aggressive control of blood pressure should be combined with optimal control of blood glucose at any stage, but most importantly when the patient manifests signs of incipient diabetic nephropathy, for it is at this point that strict metabolic control may arrest the progression of renal injury. If nonpharmacologic measures such as weight loss, exercise, and sodium restriction do not control blood pressure, then antihypertensive drug treatment should be instituted. When devising a therapeutic regimen, the clinician must consider effects on metabolic control of diabetes and cardiovascular risk factors, in addition to efficacy in control of blood pressure. In practice, a combination of drugs is often needed in diabetics with hypertension. As discussed above, the converting-enzyme inhibitors may emerge as the drugs of choice in these patients. A large clinical experience indicates that β-adrenergic blockers may be used safely in diabetics, although it seems prudent to use β_1-selective agents. If diuretics are needed, either for control of blood pressure or edema, their use should be combined with frequent monitoring for potential adverse metabolic effects, such as hyperglycemia, hypokalemia, and hyperlipidemia.

Chapter VIII

Implications of Recent Data for the Treatment of Hypertension

Norman K. Hollenberg, MD, PhD

INTRODUCTION

The goal of this chapter is to bring together the elements of what has preceded and to weave them into a workable scheme, a rational approach to the treatment of hypertension.

WHOM TO TREAT?

The more severe the hypertension, the easier is the decision to undertake medical treatment. The rationale is evident in the information from four placebo-controlled trials on the treatment of hypertension summarized in Table I. In the first Veterans Administration (VA) Cooperative trial, which involved the treatment of patients with the diastolic blood pressures ranging from 115 mm Hg to 129 mm Hg, the morbid event rate per hundred patient years was 30 in the placebo group and 2 in the treatment group (VA Cooperative Study Group, 1967). In other words, a physician would treat 100 patients per year to prevent morbid events in 28. That is very high-yield preventative therapy. In less than two years, more than half of the untreated patients would have suffered an important morbid event. In the next VA Cooperative trial, in patients with diastolic blood pressure ranging from 105 mm Hg to 114 mm Hg, the yield was lower. One would treat 100 patients for a year to improve 7 (VA Cooperative Study Group, 1970). Still, the decision is easy. Everyone agrees that a patient in whom the diastolic pressure generally exceeds 105 mm Hg merits treatment.

In the two other studies listed, the Australian trial (Report by the Management Committee, 1980) and the British Medical Research Council (MRC) trial (MRC Working Party, 1985), milder hypertension was treated, although diastolic pressures up to 105 mm Hg were included. Because milder hypertension is much more common, both studies were dominated by patients in whom the hypertension was truly mild. One has to treat large numbers of patients each year to benefit a very small number, making the decision more difficult. Note that the therapeutic impact was reduced fourfold when the lowest diastolic blood pressure criterion for entry was reduced from 95 mm Hg to 90 mm Hg.

Table I. **Benefit of treating hypertension from placebo-controlled trials.**

Study	Diastolic blood pressure (mm Hg)	Benefit/100 patient years[a]
VA Cooperative Study Group, 1967	114–129	28
VA Cooperative Study Group, 1970	105–114	7
Report by the Management Committee (Australian trial), 1980	95–104	0.48
MRC Working Party, 1985	90–104	0.12

[a] Morbid event per 100 patient years.

There is still debate on when to treat mild hypertension, especially on whether to treat diastolic blood pressures in the low 90s with drugs. The decision to undertake treatment is predicated on the answer to several questions. How confident are you that the patient indeed has hypertension? In most studies, a diastolic pressure exceeding 90 mm Hg on three separate occasions is demanded for entry, and yet 30% to 40% of the placebo-treated patients turn out not to be hypertensive. The higher the pressure is on multiple occasions, the more confident the physician should be that hypertension is present. Normotensive individuals, when they find themselves in a stressful situation, may increase their diastolic blood pressure to 110 mm Hg, and for many, a visit to a physician's office is stressful.

If on multiple examinations, at least three, the patient's diastolic blood pressure exceeds 100 mm Hg, most would agree that drug treatment is indicated. The closer the diastolic blood pressure is to 90 mm Hg, the more determinations and the longer time should be allowed before such a judgment.

The second factor determining whether drug therapy is indicated involves the other problems the patient has. Hence, in part, the focus on multifactorial elements in this book. If a person has a strong family history of hypertension, early cardiovascular events in parents and other family members, obesity, hyperlipidemia, and diabetes mellitus, is a cigarette user, or has any evidence of end-organ damage, the likelihood that one should treat rises sharply. The initial evaluation should be made with this fact in mind. As pointed out by Dr. Kaplan in Chapter II, the risk factors for atherosclerosis and coronary artery disease are more than additive, so that the impact of even mild hypertension is amplified.

THE EVALUATION OF THE PATIENT WITH HYPERTENSION

One important element in the history is a systematic review of the risk factors for coronary heart disease. Important historical factors include the use of the birth control pill, other drugs, such as prostaglandin synthetase inhibitors or nasal decongestants, a history suggestive of kidney disease or pheochromocytoma, and a review of situations in which blood pressure may have been taken earlier in other physicians' offices, for insurance or preemployment physicals, the army, and other situations.

Emphasis during the physical examination is given to evaluation of the fundi, the size of the heart, the state of the peripheral vasculature, search for an auscultatory bruit with a high-pitched systolic and diastolic component in the upper abdomen, indicative of renal artery stenosis, and stigmata suggestive of Cushing's syndrome. Particularly in the younger individual, evidence of coarctation of the aorta should be sought.

There has been substantial debate about how much laboratory evaluation is appropriate. Everyone agrees that a baseline fasting blood sugar, lipid profile, blood urea nitrogen, creatinine, serum uric acid, and serum electrolyte determination, a urinalysis, and an electrocardiogram are mandatory. With the advent of autoanalyzer testing, some of the debate on the chemical tests has softened.

Unless the person has severe hypertension, another indication of renal involvement such as a bruit, or hypertension that has been resistant to medical treatment, additional tests in search of secondary hypertension, such as the intravenous pyelogram, urine tests for pheochromocytoma, Cushing's syndrome, primary aldosteronism, renin profiling, or arteriography are generally not employed. If the hypertension is severe, complicated by other problems such as angina pectoris, congestive heart failure, or renal failure, the approach to diagnostic evaluation becomes much more aggressive.

ANTIHYPERTENSIVE TRIALS AND CORONARY ARTERY DISEASE

One might ask why has so much attention been given to risk factors for coronary artery disease and other manifestations of atherosclerosis in a book that deals primarily with converting-enzyme inhibition and the treatment of high blood pressure? The answer to that question is important, as reducing the likelihood of a coronary event is our next great challenge in the treatment of hypertension.

We have learned a great deal from a series of therapeutic trials. In one respect, our experience with antihypertensive trials has to be considered one of the great therapeutic successes of the past two decades. Clear evidence is available that therapy, whatever treatment is chosen, reduces strikingly the frequency of congestive heart failure, stroke, renal failure, accelerated hypertension, neuroretinopathy, and dissecting aneurysm. Because these complications represented a substantial fraction of the expression of high blood pressure, the result has been a clear change in natural history.

In contrast, there is an important area in which the results of treating high blood pressure have not been good. Events related to atherosclerosis, especially coronary artery disease, did not respond to the antihypertensive therapy in the same controlled trials that showed a clear benefit for heart failure, stroke, and other cardiovascular disease. Why should this be?

137

Several explanations are available. One possibility, cited by many, is that the anti-hypertensive agents used may have caused secondary effects that offset the benefits of lowering blood pressure. The most promising clue for some investigators involved the unfavorable changes in plasma lipids induced by diuretics and at least some β-blockers. There is circumstantial evidence to support this possibility, but my own suspicion is that these changes are largely transient and quantitatively not very important. Other actions of the agents used may have contributed to morbidity and mortality. One outstanding example is diuretic-induced hypokalemia, as reviewed by Dr. Kaplan in Chapter II.

Atherosclerotic events are multifactorial, involving many risk factors, and have been given special emphasis in this book. We know, on the basis of compelling evidence from many epidemiological studies, that the presence of multiple risk factors increases the likelihood of coronary artery disease in a way that is more than additive (see Chapter II). We also know that atherosclerosis, although it expresses itself clinically rather late in life in most individuals, in fact is a lifelong process. The footprints of the process can be seen in teenagers, and it is now clear that the risk factors indeed express themselves this early (Freedman et al, 1986). A second possibility to account for the failure of the antihypertensive trials to reduce coronary events reflects their focus on controlling blood pressure alone. The effort may have been too little, and too late, to reverse the vascular abnormality and prevent myocardial infarction and sudden death. The Multiple Risk Factor Intervention Trial (MRFIT; MRFIT Research Group, 1985), of course, was developed to assess this possibility. Unfortunately, despite the expenditure of vast resources, it failed to provide a clear answer. The probable explanation lies in what was happening in the community at that time. In a trial that was designed to extend over many years, creating a stable control group was impossible. The comparison group in that trial, presumably because of changes in the social milieu—prompted at least in part by our educational programs—accomplished what the treatment group did. They reduced their blood pressure, intake of saturated fats and serum cholesterol fell, and they reduced their cigarette use. As a consequence, probably both the treatment and the comparison group showed a sharp and progressive reduction in morbid events.

APPLICATION OF MULTIFACTORIAL RISK FACTOR REDUCTION

The growing recognition that the pathogenesis of coronary artery disease is multifactorial has made it clear that we must deal with more risk factors than hypertension alone to influence coronary artery disease. How shall we use the information in this book, especially that provided by Dr. Eliot and Dr. Morales-Ballejo in Chapter III?

An offhand instruction to a person, especially a new patient, that he or she should lose weight, stop eating saturated fats and replace them with fish, reduce his or her sodium intake strikingly, stop smoking, stop drinking excessive amounts of ethanol, exercise more regularly, and avoid stress is not only unlikely to be helpful, it can be counterproductive. How often today does one meet patients who are overweight and who have not already tried to lose weight? How many do not know about cholesterol or the medical cost of cigarette smoking?

How many have not already told themselves, many times, that they really must get more exercise? If a physician groups the risk factors in history taking and asks pointed questions about early death from heart disease or other complications of high blood pressure in close family members and symptoms related to heart disease in the patient, the effect is to communicate one's attitudes on these subjects without giving a lecture or sermon. It is not difficult to ascertain how ready the individual is to make the investment necessary in changing his or her behavior. The most common motivating factor, in my experience, is an early death or early stroke in a parent or sibling.

The next step involves making a clinical decision about the major problem. In the obese individual with *severe* hypertension, for example, it obviously makes little sense to attempt to correct the blood pressure problem through treatment of obesity. The blood pressure problem requires correction now; the other matters can wait. In contrast, when the individual is morbidly obese and has *mild* hypertension—if he or she seems ready to deal with the obesity—it makes excellent sense to begin with the obesity, as suggested by Dr. Eliot and Dr. Morales-Ballejo in Chapter III. For any attempt to change lifestyle to be effective, a reasonable set of goals, a useful set of guidelines, and a strong support system are required.

For most patients, attempts to modify lifestyle are part of the treatment and not the treatment itself for their high blood pressure. If the individual with hypertension is a new patient in one's practice, it makes excellent sense to get the blood pressure under control, focusing on that problem while gently letting the patient know that you will be getting to the other problems later. Once a patient has been part of one's practice for some time and success has been achieved in dealing with at least one of his or her problems, the likelihood of correcting other problems is improved. If one has achieved the obese patient's goal blood pressure with a well-tolerated drug regimen, for example, he or she can be informed that the dose of the antihypertensive agents can be reduced or even discontinued with substantial and sustained weight loss.

Although it is attractive to deal with one problem at a time, there are situations in which this is impossible. The use of diet without an exercise program is unlikely to result in substantial and sustained weight loss. In the overweight individual who has an alcohol problem, the likelihood of his or her losing weight is essentially zero unless the concomitant alcohol problem is dealt with as well.

The importance of selecting an antihypertensive agent that does not interfere with physical activity and does not compromise overall well being is highlighted by Dr. Weber and Dr. Graettinger in Chapter IV. Whether the patient's problem is obesity or peripheral vascular disease, part of the therapeutic strategy involves progressive physical activity. It makes little sense to provide instruction and encouragement on physical activity and then prescribe an agent that sharply limits physical activity. The β-adrenergic blocking agents are most troublesome in this regard. When physical activity is important, the decision to use a β-adrenergic blocking agent should be examined carefully.

139

THE SELECTION OF DRUGS FOR THE TREATMENT OF HYPERTENSION

We have today a wide range of choices for the treatment of high blood pressure. As in every other walk of life, when a series of options is available to us, the result is both an opportunity and the potential for confusion. The history of antihypertensive therapy over the past several decades is described by Dr. Materson in Chapter I. The most widely employed first-step agents for the treatment of hypertension today are the thiazide diuretics and the β-adrenergic blocking agents, and these two classes of agent were recommended by the Joint National Committee (1984) as first-step therapy. Whether their wide use reflects that Committee's recommendations or whether the Committee had responded to what had occurred in the community is not clear. What is clear is that they are widely used.

The thiazide diuretics were the wonder drugs of the late 1950s and early 1960s. Their convenience, efficacy, and safety—at least in the short run—resulted in their status as a first-step treatment. The antihypertensive properties of β-adrenergic blocking agents were not recognized until the late 1960s, and their role in antihypertensive therapy did not become dominant until the late 1970s. What prompted the move of the β-blockers?

By 1980, it had become apparent from the results of a series of placebo-controlled trials for the treatment of hypertension that the treatment regimens employed were not reducing the frequency of coronary events, either myocardial infarction or sudden death. During that time, a series of studies had documented the efficacy of β-adrenergic blockade in reducing the frequency of myocardial infarction and sudden death when used in patients after a first myocardial infarction. This series of studies on "secondary prevention" mandated the use of the β-adrenergic blocking agent in the patient at risk of myocardial infarction because of a first myocardial infarction if no contraindication for β-blockade existed. What would have been more sensible than to apply the lessons learned from secondary prevention to the problem of primary convention? Did it not make sense to utilize the β-adrenergic blocking agent for primary prevention as well?

Two trials published in 1985 provide insight into the use of thiazide diuretics and β-adrenergic blocking agents as the treatment of hypertension, with specific emphasis on coronary events.

The MRC trial involved more than 17,000 patients with mild to moderate hypertension treated for more than 85,000 patient years with either a thiazide or the β-blocker, propranolol (MRC Working Party, 1985). The size of the trial and its rigor allow us to draw definite conclusions. There was no influence of propranolol on the frequency of myocardial infarction in women. In men, an influence, and modest at that, was seen only in nonsmokers. In male smokers, the frequency of myocardial infarction was actually slightly higher when treated with propranolol, although that was not close to statistical significance. An analysis based on separation by gender and smoking habit was not part of the original working hypothesis, and so all of the weakness of a post hoc analysis is involved in this aspect of the study. On the other hand, the fact that another very large multicenter European trial, the International Prospective Primary Prevention Study in Hypertension (IPPPSH), also showed a favorable influence of β-

blockers in nonsmokers, but not in smokers does provide support for this notion (IPPPSH Collaborative Group, 1985).

Does this mean that we should choose different treatments for smokers and nonsmokers? I think not. What it does mean is that we have to pay more attention to all of the risk factors when we treat high blood pressure; the findings merely reinforce the earlier statement. The risk factors as a whole are important. The negative impact of cigarette smoking is too substantial to be overcome by β-adrenergic blockade or probably any drug regimen.

The second major trial published in 1985 with important implications for the treatment of high blood pressure was the report of the European Working Party trial on the treatment of hypertension in the elderly (Amery et al, 1985). This is the first study, I believe, to provide convincing evidence that one could reduce *mortality* in patients suffering a myocardial infarction, although the frequency of myocardial infarction was not reduced. Details of that therapeutic trial are important. This is the first trial in which a thiazide diuretic was used along with a potassium-sparing agent, triamterene. Although methyldopa was also given to about one-third of the patients, it has been used in the past without evidence of a salutary effect on mortality from myocardial infarction (Helgeland, 1980).

Why the emphasis on the potassium-sparing aspect? Certainly the entire question of the importance of potassium — and less often cited, the importance of magnesium — remains controversial. I believe that we now have enough evidence that the controversy should stop. A host of studies has now documented clearly that individuals suffering a myocardial infarction are at much greater risk of significant ventricular arrhythmias if they are hypokalemic when they reach the hospital, as reviewed by Dr. Kaplan in Chapter II. Although the studies vary in their quality and their power, there are *no* exceptions: every study has documented this fact. I agree with Dr. Kaplan's comments in Chapter II that this issue is important. To ignore the potassium and magnesium problem when employing a thiazide is to place our patients in jeopardy.

These studies have important implications for the selection of treatment. We are no longer today in a situation in which we should, or will, routinely begin treatment with either a thiazide diuretic or a β-adrenergic blocking agent for the treatment of hypertension. These agents clearly still have a place, but the selection is created in a new context.

In the case of the β-adrenergic blocking agent, the broad hope that one can reduce the likelihood of myocardial infarction is no longer tenable. When should we consider a β-adrenergic blocking agent? In the patient being treated for hypertension following myocardial infarction or with angina pectoris of effort, this class of agent is a good choice. Similarly, in the patient who has associated conditions that benefit from β-adrenergic blockade, such as migraine headache, certain forms of tremor, or hyperthyroidism, the use of a β-adrenergic blocking agent is attractive. There is a subset of very young patients with hypertension, typically under 30 years of age, in whom circulation is hyperkinetic, with a resulting tachycardia and with complaints of anxiety, palpitations, and severe anxiety under some conditions. Presumably because many of these symptoms and signs are mediated through the action of catecholamines on β-adrenergic receptors, such individuals often respond dramatically to very low doses of β-adrenergic blocking agent. Not only is their blood pressure controlled with very low doses, the dose is sufficiently low that physical activity does not seem to be limited. Their other complaints (ie, anxiety, palpitations) also are often controlled nicely.

Thiazide diuretics still have an important role in the treatment of hypertension and are likely to for some time. Indeed, whether one wants to use them or not, about 50% of the time, one is likely to find their use to be necessary if hypertension is to be controlled. Several lessons have emerged on how to use the thiazides. First, the dose should be kept low, with an initial dose of 25 mg and a top dose of 50 mg, using hydrochlorothiazide as an example. Higher doses produce progressively more electrolyte disarray, with little further gain in blood pressure control. Second, unless one is absolutely confident that the diet is adequate and will continue to be adequate and that the individual is not at risk of a coronary event, the electrolyte disarray that frequently accompanies thiazide use should be prevented. That is done most effectively by combining the thiazide with either a potassium-sparing diuretic agent or with a converting-enzyme inhibitor. The effectiveness of a converting-enzyme inhibitor reflects prevention of secondary aldosteronism. Because of the risk of hyperkalemia, a potassium-sparing agent or potassium-sparing supplement should rarely be used along with a converting-enzyme inhibitor.

CONCOMITANT ILLNESS AND DRUG SELECTION

One determinant that should shape antihypertensive therapy and is generally given too little attention has received substantial attention in this book. Concomitant illness often represents an indication or contraindication to the use of one agent or another. Positive indications for the use of β-adrenergic blocking agents were already described. Related concomitant drug use can also shape antihypertensive therapy and occurs frequently (Materson, 1985c). Dr. Materson's analysis, based on information from marketing studies, revealed that more than 50% of individuals being treated for high blood pressure had a concomitant illness or concomitant drug use that should have influenced treatment. There was no mention of the age of the individuals in Dr. Materson's analysis, and presumably a very wide age spectrum was represented. Although the frequency of hypertension in the elderly seems surprising, perhaps unbelievable, Dr. Anderson and colleagues' study of elderly individuals provides strong support to Dr. Materson's conclusions (Anderson et al, 1982). Indeed, the frequency in the elderly was substantially higher.

Dr. Case in Chapter VI reviews a substantial number of special situations created by specific clinical problems and how they might shape antihypertensive therapy. He also includes a useful review on the side-effect profile of the various antihypertensive agents available.

A substantial number of patients with hypertension also have chronic obstructive pulmonary disease or asthma, peripheral vascular disease, heart block, a history of sexual difficulties with commonly employed antihypertensive therapy, or a history of frank depression. Many others would like to maintain an active physical life and are being urged to do so by their physicians. For many, a clear sensorium free of the central nervous system side effects of commonly employed antihypertensives is important. Certainly, anyone whose livelihood depends on making judgments finds the central nervous system side effects of many antihypertensives to be unattractive. In such patients, the use of a converting-enzyme inhibitor as the mainstay of antihypertensive therapy is attractive. The combination of a low dose of a converting-enzyme inhibitor and a low dose of a thiazide diuretic is not only attractive pharmacologically, it reduces the cost to the patient and in many provides a virtual guarantee of 24-hour blood pressure control with a single daily treatment.

KEEPING PATIENTS IN TREATMENT

As we treat milder hypertension, our treatment goals must evolve. Physicians would like to provide as normal a lifestyle as possible with any treatment and for any condition. As we treat milder hypertension with antihypertensive agents, the importance of minimizing the impact of treatment on the quality of life has increased. The smaller the potential gain, the more likely it is that an individual being treated will leave treatment if annoying side effects occur. Indeed, dropouts from therapy for high blood pressure continue to be a major problem in formal trials (Curb et al, 1985a). Withdrawal from treatment in the setting of the physician's office is likely to be higher because a formal study's budget includes support personnel whose major responsibility is to call patients, find them, and get them to the clinic. How else could one sustain a study? Despite those resources, the dropout rates in major studies have been in the neighborhood of 20% in active treatment groups (Curb et al, 1985a; MRC Working Party, 1985). The number of individuals in surveys who know that they are hypertensive but remain out of treatment is substantially higher than 20% (Kaplan, 1986a). Surely, the erosion of quality of life by antihypertensive therapy must be one of the reasons that individuals leave treatment: the dropout rate in the placebo group in the MRC trial was only about 5% (MRC Working Party, 1981).

Another factor that sometimes contributes to withdrawal from treatment is cost. This seemingly simple principle finds surprising (at least surprising to me) denial from multiple sources, including both physicians and marketing people. Physicians who deny it tend to practice in the "tonier" parts of their city, and my suspicion is that their patients are well-to-do. For many individuals, it is intuitively obvious that cost must be more of a factor. Indeed, a recent poll suggests that the cost of treatment has been a major factor for 50% of individuals treated for high blood pressure. Not surprisingly, socioeconomic and racial factors appear to play a role (Gallup and Cotugno, 1986).

143

WHERE ARE WE GOING?

One of the most interesting things to do as a new treatment matures is to examine its track record from the perspective of what might have been anticipated and what could not have been anticipated. Converting-enzyme inhibition, viewed in this context, has been especially interesting. One might have anticipated that these agents would have been very useful in the patient with high renin hypertension or renovascular hypertension and in heart failure, with or without hypertension. Certainly, they have fulfilled that promise. More intriguing, at least to me, is what might never have been anticipated. In the patient with kidney disease, for example, one might have anticipated that treatment with a converting-enzyme inhibitor would have controlled the blood pressure in many, as was the case. One might have anticipated, moreover, that an agent excreted by the kidney would show an increased frequency of side effects in azotemic patients, especially when very large doses were given (Jenkins et al, 1985). This, too, was the case. What could *not* have been anticipated is that these agents might have a salutary influence on the kidney, to change natural history—slowing or preventing the progression of intrinsic renal disease, as reviewed by Dr. Raij and Dr. Tolins in Chapter VII. Circumstantial evidence in man (Thurm and Alexander, 1984) strongly supported by a large number of animal studies suggests that this might be the case; clinical studies designed to provide a definite answer are now underway.

In congestive heart failure, one might have anticipated that the reduction in preload and afterload would provide some relief. One might also have anticipated that the improvement in kidney perfusion consequent to blocking angiotensin's local action would enhance the ability of the kidney to handle salt and water and improve its overall function. This has found strong support in many clinical studies, provided that blood pressure does not fall too low (Dzau et al, 1980).

On the other hand, who could have anticipated that converting-enzyme inhibition might change the natural history of heart disease? Recent evidence from clinical studies in heart failure suggests this strongly (The CONSENSUS Trial Study Group, 1987; Furberg and Yusuf, 1985). Especially intriguing are the observations from laboratory models to suggest that converting-enzyme inhibition might modify the natural history strikingly, preventing progression of the heart disease (Pfeffer et al, 1985a, 1985b). Again, clinical studies are now underway to provide a rigorous answer to this question.

Finally, one could not have anticipated that converting-enzyme inhibition would have been effective in about 50% of patients with normal renin essential hypertension despite their use of an essentially unrestricted sodium intake (Materson, 1984). Indeed, in a dosage trial performed in Japan where sodium intake is likely to have been very high, the agent was more effective than propranolol (Kaneko et al, 1982). There are studies to suggest that converting-enzyme inhibition is effective in this setting because of an action on the renal blood supply and renal aldosterone release that facilitates sodium handling (Rystedt et al, 1986). Without the development of converting-enzyme inhibition, the critical evidence required to support this interesting possibility could not have been developed.

We may be emerging from the time in which an empirical approach is all that we have to offer most hypertensive patients. This could be the most intriguing and most important contribution of converting-enzyme inhibition in the long run.

MECHANISMS AND CHOICE OF ANTIHYPERTENSIVE THERAPY

We have been forced to choose treatment for high blood pressure to date on some basis other than the specific mechanisms involved in the individual's pathogenesis of the elevated blood pressure. Blood pressure is one of the three vital signs, along with the pulse and temperature. I find it useful to compare the approach to treatment in three areas, sepsis, arrhythmias, and hypertension.

Imagine for the moment a world in which fever was recognized but microbes and other vectors of infectious disease had not yet been identified; culture and sensitivity were not available; but yet we had discovered through empirical means some chemicals that provided a clinical benefit. It is unlikely that we would call them antibiotics. How would we choose which of these chemicals to use in an individual patient with fever? We could use the clinical story and the level and pattern of fever: individuals with a history of night sweats, chronic wasting and weight loss, cough and hemoptysis would respond to a different chemical than the individual with nocturia, urinary urgency, frequency, and dysuria. We could treat with some success, but the results would not be as good as we achieve—and expect—today. Imagine, next, that we could recognize irregularities of the pulse but that cardiac electrophysiology had not been developed and there was no electrocardiogram. We could have identified chemicals that regulated the pulse and could develop reasonable schemes for using different chemicals for different qualities of pulse, but they would not be as good as the electrocardiogram, electrophysiological studies, and Holter monitoring. Indeed, the treatment of arrhythmias with digitalis, especially atrial fibrillation, far antedated the discovery of the electrocardiogram.

We are in that situation today in the treatment of high blood pressure. We rarely treat a fundamental mechanism unless we recognize a pheochrocytoma, Cushing's syndrome, primary aldosteronism, or renovascular hypertension, and these are uncommon. Many of the strategies developed for the treatment of high blood pressure simply reflect the empiricism necessitated by our ignorance. If we could choose treatment by mechanism, the Joint National Committee's attempt to provide guidelines via "step therapy" would never have been necessary. When these guidelines were first developed in the early 1970s, they represented an attempt by the Committee to produce some order out of the chaos that was evolving, as pointed out by Dr. Materson in Chapter I. That contribution was useful at that time but, I believe, is much less useful today. We are in a position to be much more selective, and the rules for making that selection are evolving—as highlighted in several chapters in this book.

References

Abbott RD, Yin Y, Reed DM, et al: Risk of stroke in male cigarette smokers. *N Engl J Med* 1986;315:717–720.

Abramson EA, Arby RA, Woeber KA: Effects of propranolol on the hormonal and metabolic responses to insulin-induced hypoglycemia. *Lancet* 1966;2:1386–1389.

Alden L: Preventive strategies in the treatment of alcohol abuse: a review and a proposal (chapter 9), in Davidson PO, Davidson SM (eds): *Behavioral Medicine: Changing Health Lifestyles.* New York, Brunner/Mazel, Publishers, 1980, pp 256–278.

Alderman MH, Melcher L, Drayer DE, et al: Increased excretion of urinary N-acetyl-β-glucosaminidase in essential hypertension and its decline with antihypertensive therapy. *N Engl J Med* 1983;309:1213–1217.

Alexander JK: Blood pressure and obesity (chapter 57), in Matarazzo JD, Weiss SM, Herd JA, et al (eds): *Behavioral Health: A Handbook of Health Enhancement and Disease Prevention.* New York, John Wiley & Sons, 1984, pp 877–886.

Amery A, Birkenhäger W, Brixko P, et al: Mortality and morbidity results from the European Working Party on High Blood Pressure in the Elderly Trial. *Lancet* 1985;1:1349–1354.

Ames RP: Negative effects of diuretic drugs on metabolic risk factors for coronary heart disease: possible alternative drug therapies. *Am J Cardiol* 1983a;51:632–638.

Ames RP: Metabolic disturbances increasing the risk of coronary heart disease during diuretic based antihypertensive therapy: lipid alterations and glucose intolerance. *Am Heart J* 1983b;106:1207–1215.

Ames RP: Coronary heart disease and the treatment of hypertension: impact of diuretics on serum lipids and glucose. *J Cardiovasc Pharmacol* 1984;6:S466–S473.

Ames RP, Hill P: Antihypertensive therapy and the risk of coronary heart disease. *J Cardiovasc Pharmacol* 1982;4(suppl 2):S206–S212.

Anavekar SN, Barter C, Adam WR, et al: A double-blind comparison of verapamil and labetalol in hypertensive patients with coexisting chronic obstructive airway disease. *J Cardiovasc Pharmacol* 1982;4:S374–S377.

Andersen AR, Christiansen JS, Andersen JK, et al: Diabetic nephropathy in Type I (insulin-dependent) diabetes: an epidemiological study. *Diabetologia* 1983;25:496–501.

Andersen B, Snorrason SP, Ragnarsson J, et al: Hydrochlorothiazide and potassium chloride in comparison with hydrochlorothiazide and amiloride in the treatment of mild hypertension. *Acta Med Scand* 1985;218:449–454.

Anderson RJ, Reed G, Kirk LM: Therapeutic considerations for elderly hypertensives. *Clin Ther* 1982;5:25–38.

Anderson S, Rennke HG, Brenner BM: Therapeutic advantage of converting enzyme inhibitors in arresting progressive renal disease associated with systemic hypertension in the rat. *J Clin Invest* 1986;77:1993–2000.

Ando K, Fujita T, Ito Y, et al: The role of renal hemodynamics in the antihypertensive effect of captopril. *Am Heart J* 1986;111:347.

Anonymous: Sex, hormones, and atherosclerosis (editorial). *Lancet* 1986;2:552–553.

Arevalo JV: Clonidine and left ventricular function in patients with arterial hypertension. *Tribuna Medica* 1983;68:29–33.

Aromaa A, Reunanen A, Pyorala K: Hypertension and mortality in diabetic and non-diabetic Finnish men. *J Hypertens* 1984;2:S205–S207.

Atlas SA, Case DB, Sealey JE, et al: Interruption of the renin angiotensin system in hypertensive patients by captopril induces sustained reduction in aldosterone secretion, potassium retention and natriuresis. *Hypertension* 1979;1:274–280.

Ausiello DA, Zusman RM: The role of calcium in the stimulation of prostaglandin synthesis by vasopressin and angiotensin II in rabbit renal medullary interstitial cells in tissue culture. *Biochem J* 1984;220:139–145.

Avorn J, Everitt DE, Weiss S: Increased antidepressant use in patients prescribed β-blockers. *JAMA* 1986;255:357–360.

Baer L, Radichevich I: Cigarette smoking in hypertensive patients. *Am J Med* 1985;78:564–568.

Bairey CN: Exercise and coronary artery disease—What should we be recommending to our patients (and ourselves)? Medical Staff Conference, University of California, San Francisco. *West J Med* 1986;144:205–211.

Barnett AH, Leslie D, Watkins PJ: Can insulin-treated diabetics be given β-adrenergic blocking drugs? *Br Med J* 1980;280:976–978.

Barret-Connor E, Criqui MH, Klauber MR, et al: Diabetes and hypertension in a community of older adults. *Am J Epidemiol* 1981;113:276–284.

Barry DI, Pauson OB, Jarden JO, et al: Effects of captopril on cerebral blood flow in normotensive and hypertensive rats. *Am J Med* 1984;76(suppl 5B):79–85.

Bass F: Invalidating tobacco (chapter 11), in Taylor RB, Ureda JR, Denham JW (eds): *Health Promotion: Principles and Clinical Applications*. Norwalk, CT, Appleton-Century-Crofts, 1982, pp 259–286.

Bauer JH: Role of angiotensin converting enzyme-inhibitors in essential and renal hypertension. *Am J Med* 1984;77(2A):43–51.

Bauer JH, Brooks CS: The long term effects of propranolol on renal function. *Am J Med* 1979;66:405–410.

Bello CT, Servy RW, Harakal C: Varying hemodynamic patterns in essential hypertension. *Am J Med Sci* 1965;250:24–35.

Bengtsson C, Blohme G, Lapidus L, et al: Do antihypertensive drugs precipitate diabetes? *Br Med J* 1984;289:1495–1497.

Benson MK, Berrill WT, Cruickshank JM, et al: A comparison of four β-adrenoreceptor antagonists in patients with asthma. *Br J Clin Pharmacol* 1978;5:415–419.

Beretta-Piccoli C, Davies DL, Boddy K, et al: Relation of arterial pressure with body sodium, body potassium and plasma potassium in essential hypertension. *Clin Sci* 1982;63:257–270.

Beretta-Piccoli C, Weidman P, DeChatel R, et al: Hypertension associated with early stage kidney disease. Complementary roles of circulating renin, the body sodium/volume state and duration of hypertension. *Am J Med* 1976;61:739–747.

Bergner M. Bobitt A, Kressel S, et al: The sickness impact profile: conceptual formulation and methodology for the development of a health status measure. *Int J Health Serv* 1976;6:393–415.

Bertoli L, Fusco M, Micallef E, et al: Treatment of essential hypertension with captopril in patients with chronic obstructive pulmonary disease. *J Hypertension* 1985;3(suppl 2): S153–S154.

Bhatnagar SK, Amain MMA, Al-Yusuf AR: Diabetogenic effects of nifedipine. *Br Med J* 1984;289:19.

Bjork S, Nyberg G, Mulec H, et al: Beneficial effects of angiotensin converting enzyme inhibition on renal function in patients with diabetic nephropathy. *Br Med J* 1986;293:771–773.

Bjorntorp P: Regional patterns of fat distribution. *Ann Intern Med* 1985;103:994–995.

Black DG, Heagerty AM, Bing RF, et al: Effects of treatment for hypertension on cerebral haemorrhage and infarction. *Br Med J* 1984;289:156–159.

Blohm G, Lager I, Lonnroth P, et al: Hypoglycemic symptoms in insulin-dependent diabetics. A prospective study of the influence of β-blockade. *Diabetes Metab* 1981;7:235–238.

Blum M, Bauminger S, Algenti A, et al: Urinary prostaglandin-E$_2$ in chronic renal disease. *Clin Nephrol* 1981;15:87–89.

Bouthier JD, De Luca N, Safar ME, et al: Cardiac hypertrophy and arterial distensibility in essential hypertension. *Am Heart J* 1985;109:1345–1352.

Breslow LA: A quantitative approach to the world health organization definition of health: physical, mental and social well-being. *Int J Epidemiol* 1972;1:347–355.

Brown LE, Ellis EO: Foreword, *Quality of Life: The Later Years.* Acton, MA, Publishing Sciences Group, Inc, 1975.

Buell JC, Eliot RS: Psychosocial and behavioral influences in the pathogenesis of acquired cardiovascular disease. *Am Heart J* 1980;100:723–740.

Bühler FR, Laragh JM, Baer L, et al: Propranolol inhibition of renin secretion: a specific approach to diagnosis and treatment of renin dependent hypertensive disease. *N Engl J Med* 1972;287:1209.

Bulpitt CJ, Dollery CT: Side effects of hypotensive agents evaluated by a self-administered questionnaire. *Br Med J* 1973;3:485–490.

Bulpitt CJ, Dollery CT, Carne S: Change in symptoms of hypertensive patients after referral to hospital clinic. *Br Heart J* 1976;38:121–128.

Burris JF, Goldstein J, Zager PG, et al: Comparative tolerability of labetalol versus propranolol, atenolol, pindolol, metoprolol, and nadolol. *J Clin Hypertens* 1986;3:285–293.

Campbell A, Converse PE, Rodger WL: *The Quality of American Life.* New York, Russel Sage Foundation, 1976, pp 1–18.

Cantril H: *The Pattern of Human Concerns.* New Brunswick, NJ, Rutgers University Press, 1965.

Caralis PV, Materson BJ, Perez-Stable EC: Potassium and diuretic-induced ventricular arrhythmias in ambulatory hypertensive patients. *Mineral Electrolyte Metab* 1984;10: 148–154.

Carr AA: Hypertension Rx: diuretic or β-blocker first? *Mod Med* 1984;52:124–131.

Casale PN, Devereux RB, Milner M, et al: Value of echocardiographic measurement of left ventricular mass in predicting cardiovascular morbid events in hypertensive men. *Ann Intern Med* 1986;105:173–178.

Case DB, Atlas SA, Marion RM, et al: Long-term efficacy of captopril in renovascular and essential hypertension. *Am J Cardiol* 1982;49:1440–1446.

Castelli WP: Epidemiology of coronary heart disease: the Framingham study. *Am J Med* 1984;76:4–12.

Castelli WP, Anderson K: A population at risk: prevalence of high cholesterol levels in hypertensive patients in the Framingham study. *Am J Med* 1986;80(suppl 2A):23–32.

Chamberlain DA, Howard J: Guanethidine and methyldopa: a hemodynamic study. *Br Heart J* 1964;26:528–536.

Charles S, Ketelslegers JM, Buysschaert M, et al: Hyperglycaemia effect of nifedipine. *Br Med J* 1981;283:19–20.

Chatel R, Weidmann P, Flammer J, et al: Sodium, renin, aldosterone, catecholamines and blood pressure in diabetes mellitus. *Kidney Int* 1977;12:412–421.

Chesney MA, Rosenman RH (eds): *Anger and Hostility in Cardiovascular and Behavioral Disorders.* Washington, DC, Hemisphere Publishing Corp, 1985.

Chiang BN, Perlman LV, Epstein FH: Overweight and hypertension: a review. *Circulation* 1969;39:403–421.

Chimori K, Miyazaki S, Kosaka J, et al: Increased sodium influx into erythrocytes in diabetes mellitus and hypertension. *Clin Exp Hypertens* 1986;8:185–199.

Christensen NJ, Brandsborg O: The relationship between plasma catecholamine concentration and pulse rate during exercise and standing. *Eur J Clin Invest* 1973;3:299–306.

Christlieb AR: Renin-angiotensin-aldosterone system in diabetes mellitus. *Diabetes* 1976;25(suppl 2):820–825.

Christlieb AR, Janka HU, Kraus B, et al: Vascular reactivity to angiotensin II and to norepinephrine in diabetes mellitus. *Diabetes* 1976a;25:268–274.

Christlieb AR, Kaldany A, D'Elia JA: Plasma renin activity and hypertension in diabetes mellitus. *Diabetes* 1976b;25:969–974.

Christlieb AR, Warren JH, Krolewski AS, et al: Hypertension: the major risk factor in juvenile onset insulin dependent diabetics. *Diabetes* 1981;30(suppl 2):90–96.

Chrysant SG, Luu TM, Danisa K, et al: Systemic and renal hemodynamic effects of trimazosin: a new vasodilator. *J Cardiovasc Pharmacol* 1980;2:205–214.

Cody RJ, Tarazi RC, Bravo EL, et al: Hemodynamics of orally-active converting enzyme inhibitor (SQ14225) in hypertensive patients. *Clin Sci Mol Med* 1978;55:453–459.

Cohen LM, Anderson G, White RF, et al: Enalapril and hypertension (letter to the editor). *Am J Psych* 1984;141(8):1012–1013.

Cohn JN, Levine TB, Francis GS, et al: Neurohumoral control mechanisms in congestive heart failure. *Am Heart J* 1981;102:509–514.

Conlon PF, Grambau GR, Johnson CE, et al: Effect of intravenous furosemide on serum theophylline concentration. *Am J Hosp Pharm* 1981;38:1345–1347.

Consensus Conference: Lowering blood cholesterol to prevent heart disease. *JAMA* 1985;253:2080–2086.

The CONSENSUS Trial Study Group: Effects of enalapril on mortality in severe congestive heart failure: results of the Cooperative North Scandinavian Enalapril Survival Study (CONSENSUS). *N Engl J Med* 1987;316:1429–1435.

Corsis PA, Nariman S, Gibson GJ: Nifedipine in the prevention of asthma induced by exercise and histamine. *Am Rev Resp Dis* 1983;128:991–992.

Creager MA, Halperin JL, Bernard DB, et al: Acute regional circulatory and renal hemodynamic effects of converting-enzyme inhibition in patients with congestive heart failure. *Circulation* 1981;64:483–489.

Croog SH, Levine S, Testa MA, et al: The effects of antihypertensive therapy on the quality of life. *N Engl J Med* 1986;314:1657–1664.

Croog SH, Sudilovsky A, Levine S, et al: Work performance, absenteeism and antihypertensive medications. *J Hypertens* 1987;5(suppl 1):S47–S54.

Curb JD, Borhani NO, Blaszkowski TP, et al: Long-term surveillance for adverse effects of antihypertensive drugs. *JAMA* 1985a;253:3263–3268.

Curb JD, Borhani NO, Blaszkowski TP, et al: Patient-perceived side effects to antihypertensive drugs. *Am J Prev Med* 1985b;1:36–40.

Dahlof B, Andren L, Eggertsen R, et al: Potentiation of the antihypertensive effect of enalapril by randomized addition of different doses of hydrochlorothiazide. *J Hypertens* 1985;3(suppl 3):S483–S486.

D'Angelo A, Sartori L, Gambaro G, et al: Captopril in the treatment of hypertension in type I and type II diabetic patients. *Postgrad Med J* 1986;62(suppl 1):69–72.

Day JL, Metcalfe J, Simpson CN: Adrenergic mechanisms in control of plasma lipid concentrations. *Br Med J* 1982;284:1145–1148.

Day JL, Metcalfe J, Simpson N, et al: Adrenergic mechanisms in the control of plasma lipids in man. *Am J Med* 1984;76:94–96.

De Fronzo RA: The effect of insulin on renal sodium metabolism: a review with clinical implications. *Diabetologia* 1981;21:165–171.

Deacon SP, Karunanayake A, Barnett D: Acebutolol, atenolol and propranolol and metabolic responses to acute hypoglycemia in diabetics. *Br J Med* 1977;2:1255–1257.

Deanfield J, Wright C, Krikler S, et al: Cigarette smoking in the treatment of angina with propranolol, atenolol, and nifedipine. *N Engl J Med* 1984;310:951–954.

Deckert T, Pouken JE, Larsen M: Prognosis of diabetics with diabetes onset before age 31. *Diabetologia* 1978;14:363–370.

deLeeuw PW, Birkenhager WH: Renal blood flow in hypertension: relationships to sodium excretion and adrenergic activity. *NZ Med J* 1983;96:851–852.

DeLeive A, Christlieb AR, Melby JC, et al: Big renin and biosynthetic defect of aldosterone in diabetes mellitus. *N Eng J Med* 1976;295:639–643.

DeMarinis L, Barbarino A: Calcium antagonists and hormone release. I. Effects of verapamil on insulin release in normal subjects and patients with islet-cell tumor. *Metabolism* 1980;29:599–604.

Deragotis LR, Spencer PM: *The Brief Symptom Inventory (BSI), Administration, Scoring and Procedures Manual I.* Baltimore, Johns Hopkins University School of Medicine (privately printed), 1982.

deWit H, Camic PM: Behavioral and pharmacological treatment of cigarette smoking: end of treatment comparisons. *Addict Behav* 1986;11:331–335.

Dhingra S, Solven F, Wilson A, et al: Hypomagnesemia and respiratory muscle power. *Am Rev Resp Dis* 1984;129:497–498.

Diakonova EG, Iurenev AP: Hemodynamic mechanism of the hypotensive action of diuretics and their effect on myocardial hypertrophy in the process of long-term treatment of hypertension. *Biull Vsesoiuznogo Kardiol Nauchn Tsentra AMN SSSR* 1982;5:57–61.

Diamond JR, Cheung JY, Fang LST: Nifedipine-induced renal dysfunction: alterations in renal hemodynamics. *Am J Med* 1984;77:905–909.

Dimsdale JE: Controversies regarding type A behavior and coronary heart disease. *Cardiology Clinics* 1985;3:259–267.

Dimsdale JE, Pierce C, Schoenfeld D, et al: Suppressed anger and blood pressure: the effects of race, sex, social class, obesity, and age. *Psychosom Med* 1986;48:430–436.

Dollery CT: The decision to treat: profiling benefit. *J Hypertens* 1985;3(suppl 2):S41–S44.

Dominguez JR, de La Calle H, Hurtado A, et al: Effect of converting enzyme inhibitors in hypertensive patients with non-insulin dependent diabetes mellitus. *Postgrad Med J* 1986;62(suppl 1):66–68.

Dornhorst A, Powell SH, Pensky J: Aggravation by propranolol of hyperglycaemic effect of hydrochlorothiazide in type II diabetics without alteration of insulin secretion. *Lancet* 1985;1:123–126.

Drayer JIM, Weber MA: Monotherapy of essential hypertension with a converting-enzyme inhibitor. *Hypertension* 1983;(suppl 3):108–113.

Drayer JIM, Gardin JM, Weber MA, et al: Changes in cardiac anatomy and function during therapy with alpha-methyldopa: an echocardiographic study. *Curr Ther Res* 1982a;32:856–865.

Drayer JIM, Gardin JM, Weber MA, et al: Changes in ventricular septal thickness during diuretic therapy. *Clin Pharmacol Ther* 1982b;32:283–288.

Drayer JIM, Weber MA, Lipson JL, et al: Different effects of diuresis and beta-adrenergic blockade during angiotensin converting enzyme inhibition in patients with severe hypertension. *J Clin Pharmacol* 1982c;22:179–186.

Dreslinski GR, Messerli FH, Dunn FG, et al: Hemodynamics, biochemical and reflexive changes produced by atenolol in hypertension. *Circulation* 1982;65:1365–1368.

DuCharme DW, Freyburger WA, Graham BE, et al: Pharmacologic properties of minoxidil: a new hypotensive agent. *J Pharmacol Exp Ther* 1973;184:662–670.

Duffy DJ, Horwitz LD, Brammell HL: Nifedipine and the conditioning response. *Am J Cardiol* 1984;53:908–912.

Duncan JH, Faris IB: Skin vascular resistance and skin perfusion pressure as predictors of healing of ischemic lesion of the lower limb: influences of diabetes mellitus, hypertension, and age. *Surgery* 1986;99:432–438.

Dupuy HJ: *Developmental Rationale, Substantive, Derivatable, and Conceptual Relevance for the General Well-Being Schedule.* Fairfax, VA, National Center for Health Statistics, 1973.

Dzau VJ: Significance of the vascular renin-angiotensin pathway. *Hypertension* 1986;8:553–559.

Dzau VJ, Colucci WS, Hollenberg NK, et al: Sustained effectiveness of converting-enzyme inhibition in patients with severe congestive heart failure. *N Engl J Med* 1980;302:1373–1379.

Editorial: Treatment of hypertension in the over-60s. *Lancet* 1985;1:1369–1370.

Ekelund LG: Nifedipine in combination therapy for chronic hypertension. *Am J Med* 1985;79(suppl 4A):41–43.

Eliot RS, Bratt G: The paradox of myocardial ischemia and necrosis in young women with normal coronary arteriograms: relation to abnormal hemoglobin-oxygen dissociation. *Am J Cardiol* 1969;23:633–638.

Eliot RS, Breo DL: *Is It Worth Dying For?* New York, Bantam Books, 1984.

Ellestad MH: Ischemic S-T segment depression: hemodynamic, electrophysiologic, and metabolic factors in its genesis, in Ellestad MH (ed): *Stress Testing: Principles and Practice* (2nd ed). Philadelphia, FA Davis Co, 1980, pp 77–96.

Engstrom D: A psychological perspective of prevention in alcoholism (chapter 72), in Matarazzo JD, Weiss SM, Herd JA, et al (eds): *Behavioral Health: A Handbook of Health Enhancement and Disease Prevention.* New York, John Wiley & Sons, 1984, pp 1047–1058.

Enos WF, Holmes RH, Beyer J: Coronary disease among United States soldiers killed in action in Korea: preliminary report. *JAMA* 1953;152:1090–1093.

Epstein LH, Jennings JR: Smoking, stress, cardiovascular reactivity and coronary heart disease (chapter 15), in Mathers KA, Weiss SM, Detre T, et al (eds): *Handbook of Stress Reactivity and Cardiovascular Disease.* New York, John Wiley & Sons, 1986, pp 291–309.

Epstein SE, Robinson BF, Kahler RL, et al: Effects of beta-adrenergic blockade on the cardiac response to maximal and submaximal exercise in man. *J Clin Invest* 1965;44:1745–1753.

Eriksen L, Bjornstad S, Gotestam KG: Social skills training in groups for alcoholics: one-year treatment outcome for groups and individuals. *Addict Behav* 1986;11:309–329.

Ewing DJ, Irving JB, Kerr F, et al: Static exercise in untreated systemic hypertension. *Br Heart J* 1973;35:413–421.

Fagard R, Lijnen P, Amery A: Hemodynamic response to captopril at rest and during exercise in hypertensive patients. *Am J Cardiol* 1982;49:1569–1571.

Fagard R, Amery A, Reybrouck T, et al: Acute and chronic systemic and pulmonary hemodynamic effects of angiotensin converting enzyme inhibition with captopril in hypertensive patients. *Am J Cardiol* 1980;46:295–300.

Falkner B, Onesti G, Hamstra B: Stress response characteristics of adolescents with high genetic risk for essential hypertension: a five year follow-up. *Clin Exp Hypertens* 1981a; 3:583–591.

Falkner B, Onesti G, Angelakos E: Effect of salt loading on the cardiovascular response to stress in adolescents. *Hypertension* 1981b;3(suppl II):II195–II199.

Falkner B, Onesti G, Angelakos ET, et al: Cardiovascular response to mental stress in normal adolescents with hypertensive parents. *Hypertension* 1979;1:23–26.

Feinstein AR: The Jones criteria and the challenges of clinimetrics. *Circulation* 1982;66:1–5.

Feinstein AR, Josephy BR, Wells CK: Scientific and clinical problems in indexes of functional disability. *Ann Intern Med* 1986;105:413–420.

Feinstein AR, Wells CK, Joyce CM, et al: The evaluation of sensibility and the role of patient collaboration in clinimetric indexes. *Trans Assoc Am Physicians* 1985;98:146–149.

Feldt-Rasmussen B, Borch-Johnsen K, Mathiesen ER: Hypertension in diabetes as related to nephropathy: early blood pressure changes. *Hypertension* 1985;7:118–120.

Feldt-Rasmussen B, Mathiesen ER, Deckert T: Effect of two years of strict metabolic control on progression of incipient nephropathy in insulin dependent diabetics. *Lancet* 1986;2:1301–1304.

Ferguson JM: Behavior modification and health care systems (chapter 5), in Taylor RB, Ureda JR, Denham JW (eds): *Health Promotion: Principles and Clinical Applications*. Norwalk, CT, Appleton-Century-Crofts, 1982, pp 123–142.

Ferrier C, Beretta-Picolli C, Weidmann P, et al: Alpha-1-adrenergic blockade and lipoprotein metabolism in essential hypertension. *Clin Pharmacol Ther* 1986;40:525–530.

Ferriere M, Lachkar H, Richard JL, et al: Captopril and insulin sensitivity. *Ann Intern Med* 1985;102:134–135.

Final Report of the Subcommittee on Nonpharmacological Therapy of the 1984 Joint National Committee on Detection, Evaluation, and Treatment of High Blood Pressure: Nonpharmacological approaches to the control of high blood pressure. *Hypertension* 1986;8:444–467.

Flamenbaum M: Metabolic consequences of antihypertensive therapy. *Ann Intern Med* 1983;98(part 2):875–880.

Fleishman AI, Bierenbaum ML, Stier A: Effect of stress due to anticipated minor surgery upon *in vivo* platelet aggregation in humans. *J Human Stress* 1976;2:33.

Fletcher GF: Cardiovascular disease primary prevention – role of exercise and other risk factor modification (chapter 4), in Fletcher GF: *Exercise in the Practice of Medicine*. Mount Kisco, NY, Futura Publishing Co, 1982, pp 103–146.

Flink EB: Magnesium deficiency: etiology and clinical spectrum. *Acta Med Scand Suppl* 1981;647:125–137.

Floras J, Hassan MO, Jones JV, et al: Contrasting effects of cardioselective and nonselective beta blockers on changes in blood pressure during bicycle exercise in subjects with essential hypertension (abstract). *J Am Cardiol* 1983;1:625.

Folkow B: Physiologic aspects of primary hypertension. *Physiological Reviews* 1982;62:347-504.

Forgoros RN: Exacerbation of intermittent claudication by propranolol (letter). *N Engl J Med* 1980;302:1089.

Franz IW, Lohmann FW, Koch G, et al: Aspects of hormonal regulation of exercise: effects of chronic beta-receptor blockade. *Int J Sports Med* 1983;4:14–20.

Freedman DS, Srinivisan SR, Shear CL, et al: The relation of apolipoproteins A-1 and B in children to parental myocardial infarction. *N Engl J Med* 1986;315:721–726.

Freestone S, Ramsay LE: Effect of coffee and cigarette smoking on the blood pressure of untreated and diuretic-treated hypertensive patients. *Am J Med* 1982;73:348–353.

Freis ED: Validity of therapy for mild hypertension. *Ann Rev Med* 1979;30:81–89.

Freis ED: Should mild hypertension be treated? *N Engl J Med* 1982;307:306–309.

Freis ED: The cardiovascular risks of thiazide diuretics. *Clin Pharmacol Ther* 1986;39:239–244.

Freis ED, Papademetriou V: Thiazides do not increase cardiovascular risk. *Drug Therapy* 1986;16:41–49.

Friedman M, Rosenman RH: Association of specific overt behavior pattern with increases in blood cholesterol, blood clotting time, incidence of arcus senilis and clinical coronary heart disease. *JAMA* 1959;169:1286–1296.

Friedman M, Thoresen CE, Gill JJ, et al: Alteration of type A behavior and its effect on cardiac recurrences in post myocardial infarction patients: summary results of the recurrent coronary prevention project. *Am Heart J* 1986;112:653–665.

Frieds JF: Aging, natural death, and the compression of morbidity. *N Engl J Med* 1980;303:130–135.

Frishman WH: β-Adrenoreceptor-antagonists: new drugs and indications. *N Engl J Med* 1981;305:500–506.

Frishman WH, Michelson EL, Johnson BF, et al: Multiclinic comparison of labetalol to metoprolol in treatment of mild to moderate systemic hypertension. *Am J Med* 1983;75(suppl 4A):54–67.

Frisk-Holmberg M, Strom G: Exercise during therapeutic beta-blockade: a two-year study in hypertensive patients. *Clin Pharmacol Ther* 1986;40:395–399.

Frisk-Holmberg M, Jorfeldt L, Juhlin-Dannfelt A: Metabolic effects in muscle during anti-hypertensive therapy with β_1 and β_2-adrenoceptor blockade. *Clin Pharmacol Ther* 1981;30:611–618.

Frisk-Holmberg M, Jorfeldt L, Juhlin-Dannfelt A, et al: Metabolic changes in muscle on long-term alprenolol therapy. *Clin Pharmacol Ther* 1979;26:566–571.

Frohlich ED, Tarazi RC: Is arterial pressure the sole factor responsible for hypertensive cardiac hypertrophy? *Am J Cardiol* 1979;44:959–963.

Frohlich ED, Tarazi RC, Dustan HP: Reexamination of the hemodynamics of hypertension. *Am J Med Sci* 1969;257:9–23.

Frohlich ED, Messerli FH, Dreslinski GR, et al: Long-term renal hemodynamic effects of nadolol in patients with essential hypertension. *Am Heart J* 1984;108:1141–1143.

Frohlich ED, Messerli FH, Reisen E, et al: The problem of obesity and hypertension. *Hypertension* 1983;5(suppl 3):71–78.

Fujitani K, Mitsuda H, Eno S, et al: Effect of SQ 14425 (captopril) on hemodynamics, plasma renin activity, plasma aldosterone concentration and plasma catecholamines in essential hypertension. *Jpn Circ J* 1979;43:711–712.

Fuller JH: Epidemiology of hypertension associated with diabetes mellitus. *Hypertension* 1985a;7:113–117.

Fuller JH: Blood pressure and diabetes (chapter 21), in Birkenhager WH, Reid JL (eds): *Epidemiology of Hypertension*. Vol 6. New York, Elsevier, 1985b, p 319.

Fuller JH, Shipley MJ, Rose G, et al: Mortality from coronary heart disease and stroke in relation to degree of glycaemia: the Whitehall study. *Br Med J* 1983;287:867–870.

Furberg CD, Yusuf S: Effects of vasodilators on survival in chronic congestive heart failure. *Am J Cardiol* 1985;55:1110–1113.

Furberg CD, Schucker MA, Chesney MA, et al: Report of the working group: mild hypertension, in Wenger NK, Mattson ME, Furberg CD, et al (eds): *Assessment of Quality of Life in Clinical Trials of Cardiovascular Therapies*. New York, Le Jacq Publishing Inc, 1984, pp 285–295.

Gallup G, Cotugno HE: Preferences and practices of Americans and their physicians in anti-hypertensive therapy. *Am J Med* 1986;81:20–24.

Garfield SR, Collen MF, Feldman R, et al: Evaluation of an ambulatory medical care delivery system. *N Engl J Med* 1976;294:426–431.

Gent AN: Fracture of elastomers, in Liebowitz H (ed): *Fracture*. New York, Academic Press, 1972.

Gerber A, Weidmann P, Bianchetti MG, et al: Serum lipoproteins during treatment with the antihypertensive agent indapamide. *Hypertension* 1985;7(suppl II):II164–II169.

Gillum RF, Taylor HL, Brozek J, et al: Indices of obesity and blood pressure in young men followed 32 years. *J Chron Dis* 1982;35:211–219.

Ginks WR, Redwood DR: Hemodynamic effects of hydralazine at rest and during exercise in patients with chronic heart failure. *Br Heart J* 1980;44:259–264.

Gokal R, Dornan TL, Ledingham JGG: Peripheral skin necrosis complicating β-blockade. *Br Med J* 1979;1:721–722.

Goldbourt U, Holtzman E, Neufeld HN: Total and high density lipoprotein cholesterol in the serum and risk of mortality: evidence of a threshold effect. *Br Med J* 1985;290:1239–1243.

Goldman L, Cook F: The decline in ischemic heart disease mortality rates. *Ann Intern Med* 1984;101:825–836.

Goldner MG, Zarowitz H, Akgun S: Hyperglycaemia and glucosuria due to thiazide derivatives administered in diabetes mellitus. *N Engl J Med* 1960;262:403–405.

Goldring W, Chasis H: Antihypertensive drug therapy: an appraisal, in Ingelfinger FJ, Relman AS, Finland M (eds): *Controversy in Internal Medicine*. Philadelphia, WB Saunders Co, 1966, p 83.

Goldstein DS: Plasma norepinephrine in essential hypertension. A study of studies. *Hypertension* 1981;3:48–52.

Goodfellow R: Proximal myopathy during beta blockade (letter). *Br Med J* 1980;280:399–400.

Gordon T, Kannel WB: Multiple risk functions for predicting coronary heart disease: the concept, accuracy, and application. *Am Heart J* 1982;103:1031–1039.

Gordon T, Kannel WB, Dawber TR, et al: Changes associated with quitting cigarette smoking: the Framingham Study. *Am Heart J* 1975;90:322–328.

Gottlieb TB, Katz FH, Chidsey CA: Combined therapy with vasodilator drugs and beta-adrenergic blockade in hypertension: a comparative study of minoxidil and hydralazine. *Circulation* 1972;45:571–582.

Gould BA, Hornung RS, Mann S: Slow channel inhibitors verapamil and nifedipine in the management of hypertension. *J Cardiovasc Pharmacol* 1982;4(suppl 3):S369–S374.

Green MS, Jucha E, Luz Y: Blood pressure in smokers and nonsmokers: epidemiologic findings. *Am Heart J* 1986;111:932–940.

Greenblatt DJ, Koch-Weser J: Adverse reactions to propranolol in hospitalized medical patients: a report from the Boston Collaborative Drug Surveillance Program. *Am Heart J* 1973;86:478–484.

Grignolo A, Koepke JP, Obrist PA: Renal function, heart rate, and blood pressure during exercise and shock avoidance in dogs. *Am J Physiol* 1982;242:R482–R490.

Grimm RH Jr, Leon AS, Hunninghake DB, et al: Effects of thiazide diuretics on plasma lipids and lipoproteins in mildly hypertensive patients. *Ann Intern Med* 1981;94:7–11.

Grogono AW, Woodgate DJ: Index for measuring health. *Lancet* 1971;1:1024–1026.

Groop L, Totterman K, Harno K, et al: Influence of beta-blocking drugs on glucose metabolism in patients with non-insulin dependent diabetes mellitus. *Acta Med Scand* 1982;211:7–12.

Grunfeld C, Chappell DA: Hypokalemia and diabetes mellitus. *Am J Med* 1983;75:553–554.

Guthrie GP, Miller RE, Kotchen TA, et al: Clonidine in patients with diabetes and mild hypertension. *Clin Pharmacol Ther* 1983;34:713–717.

Haft JI, Arkel YS: Effect of emotional stress on platelet aggregation in humans. *Chest* 1976;70:501.

Halperin AK, Cubeddu LX: The role of calcium channel blockers in the treatment of hypertension. *Am Heart J* 1986;111:363–382.

Hammond IW, Devereux RB, Alderman MH, et al: The prevalence and correlates of echocardiographic left ventricular hypertrophy among employed patients with uncomplicated hypertension. *J Am Coll Cardiol* 1986;7:639–650.

Hannson L: Hemodynamic effects of acute and prolonged beta-adrenergic blockade in essential hypertension (abstract). *Scand J Clin Lab Invest* 1975;35(suppl 143):59.

Harburg E, Erfurt J, Hauenstein L, et al: Socioecological stress, suppressed hostility, skin color, and black-white male blood pressure: Detroit. *Psychosom Med* 1973;35:276–296.

Hardy RJ, Hawkins CM: The impact of selected indices of antihypertensive treatment on all-cause mortality. *Am J Epidemiol* 1983;117:566–574.

Hare TW, Lowenthal DT, Hakki HH, et al: The effect of exercise training in older patients on beta adrenergic blocking drugs. *Ann Sports Med* 1984.

Harvald B: The hypertensive genotype. *Scand J Prim Health Care* 1984;3:96–97.

Haynes RB, Mattson ME, Chobanian AV, et al: Management of patient compliance in the treatment of hypertension. Report of the NHLBI Working Group. *Hypertension* 1982;4:415–423.

Haynes RB, Sackett DL, Taylor DW, et al: Increased absenteeism from work after detection and labeling of hypertensive patients. *N Engl J Med* 1978;299:741–744.

Heel RC, Brogden RN, Speight TM, et al: Captopril: a preliminary review of its pharmacologic properties and therapeutic efficacy. *Drugs* 1980;20:409–452.

Helderman JH, Elahi D, Andersen DK, et al: Prevention of glucose intolerance of thiazide diuretics by maintenance of body potassium. *Diabetes* 1983;32:106–111.

Helgeland A: Treatment of mild hypertension: a 5-year controlled drug trial. The Oslo Study. *Am J Med* 1980;69:725–732.

Heller RF, Chinn S, Tunstall Pedoe HD, et al: How well can we predict coronary heart disease? Findings in the United Kingdom heart disease prevention project. *Br Med J* 1984;288:1409–1411.

Henderson BE, Ross RK, Pagnini-Hill A, et al: Estrogen use and cardiovascular disease. *Am J Obstet Gynecol* 1986;154:1181–1186.

Henningsen NC: Hypertension and the use of diabetogenic diuretics. *Acta Pharmacol Toxicol* 1984;54(suppl 1):71–73.

Henry JP, Ely DL: Physiology of emotional stress: specific responses. *J South Carolina Med Assoc* 1979;75:501–509.

Herold PM, Kinsella JE: Fish oil consumption and decreased risk of cardiovascular disease: a comparison of findings from animal and human feeding trials. *Am J Clin Nutr* 1986; 43:566–598.

Heyden S: The Workingman's diet. II. Effect of weight reduction in obese patients with hypertension, diabetes, hyperuricemia and hyperlipidemia. *Nutr Metab* 1978;22:141–159.

Heyden S, Bartel AG, Hames CG, et al: Elevated blood pressure levels in adolescents, Evans County, Georgia: seven-year follow-up of 30 patients and 30 controls. *JAMA* 1969;209: 1683–1689.

Heyden S, Cassel JC, Bartel A, et al: Body weight and cigarette smoking as risk factors. *Arch Intern Med* 1971;128:915–919.

Hill JF, Bulpitt CJ, Fletcher AE: Angiotensin-converting enzyme inhibitors and quality of life: the European trial. *J Hypertens* 1985;3(suppl 2):S91–S94.

Hill NS: Fluid and electrolyte considerations in diuretic therapy for hypertensive patients with chronic obstructive pulmonary disease. *Arch Intern Med* 1986;146:129–133.

Hofman A, Roelandt JTRC, Boomsma F, et al: Hemodynamics, plasma noradrenaline, and plasma renin in hypertensive and normotensive teenagers. *Clin Sci* 1981;61:169–174.

Hohnloser SH, Verrier RL, Lown B, et al: Effect of hypokalemia on susceptibility to ventricular fibrillation in the normal and ischemic canine heart. *Am Heart J* 1986;112:32–35.

Hollenberg NK: When should mild essential hypertension be treated? *Drug Ther* 1982;12:65–67.

Hollenberg NK, Borucki LJ, Adams DF: The renal vasculature in early essential hypertension: evidence for a pathogenic role. *Medicine* 1978;57:167–178.

Hollenberg NK, Williams GH, Adams DF: Essential hypertension: abnormal renal vascular and endocrine responses to a mild psychological stimulus. *Hypertension* 1981;3:11–17.

Hollenberg NK, Adams DF, McKinstry DN, et al: Beta-adrenoceptor-blocking agents and the kidney: effect of nadolol and propranolol on the renal circulation. *Br J Clin Pharmacol* 1979;7(suppl 2):219–223.

Hollifield JW: Potassium and magnesium abnormalities: diuretics and arrhythmias in hypertension. *Am J Med* 1984;77:28–32.

Holme I, Helgeland A, Hjermann I, et al: Treatment of mild hypertension with diuretics: the importance of ECG abnormalities in the Oslo Study and in MRFIT. *JAMA* 1984;251: 1298–1299.

Hommel E, Parving HH, Mathiesen E, et al: Effect of captopril on kidney function in insulin-dependent diabetic patients with nephropathy. *B Med J* 1986;293:467–470.

Hostetter TH: Pathogenesis of diabetic nephropathy (chapter 9), in Brenner B, Stein J (eds): *The Progressive Nature of Renal Disease.* Edinburgh, Churchill Livingston, 1986, pp 149–166.

Hostetter TH, Rennke HG, Brenner BM: The case of intrarenal hypertension in the initiation and progression of diabetic and other glomerulopathies. *Am J Med* 1982;72:375–380.

Hricik DE, Browning PJ, Kopelman R, et al: Captopril-induced functional renal insufficiency in patients with bilateral renal-artery stenoses or renal artery stenosis in a solitary kidney. *N Engl J Med* 1983;308:373–376.

Hubert H, Feinleib M, McNamara P, et al: Obesity as an independent risk factor for cardiovascular disease: a 26-year follow-up of participants in the Framingham heart study. *Circulation* 1983;67:968–977.

Hunt JC, Sheps SG, Harrison EG, et al: Renal and renovascular hypertension. A reasoned approach to diagnosis and management. *Arch Intern Med* 1974;133:988–999.

Hurtig HI, Dyson WL: Lithium toxicity enhanced by diuresis (letter). *N Engl J Med* 1974;290:748–749.

Hypertension Detection and Follow-up Program Cooperative Group: The hypertension detection and follow-up program: a progress report. *Circ Res* 1977;40(suppl 1):106–109.

Hypertension Detection and Follow-up Program Cooperative Group: Five-year findings of the hypertension detection and follow-up program. I. Reduction in mortality of persons with high blood pressure, including mild hypertension. *JAMA* 1979a;242:2562–2571.

Hypertension Detection and Follow-up Program Cooperative Group: Five-year findings of the hypertension detection and follow-up program. II. Mortality by race, sex and age. *JAMA* 1979b;242:2572–2577.

Hypertension Detection and Follow-up Program Cooperative Group: Five-year findings of the hypertension detection and follow-up program. III. Reduction and stroke incidence among persons with high blood pressure. *JAMA* 1982;247:633–638.

Ingram DM, House AK, Thompson GH, et al: Beta adrenergic blockade and peripheral vascular disease. *Med J Aust* 1982;1:509–511.

International Collaborative Group: International collaborative study on juvenile hypertension. 2. First follow-up report. *Bulletin of World Health Org* 1984;62:121–132.

The IPPPSH Collaborative Group: Cardiovascular risks and risk factors in a randomized trial of treatment based on the β-blocker oxprenolol: the International Prospective Primary Prevention Study in Hypertension (IPPPSH) *Hypertension* 1985;3:379-392.

Isles C: Excess smoking in malignant hypertension. *Am Heart J* 1980;99:538–539.

Jachuck SJ, Brierley H, Jachuck S, et al: The effect of hypotensive drugs on the quality of life. *J Royal Coll Gen Pract* 1982;32:103–105.

Jarvis MJ, Raw M, Russell MAH, et al: Randomized controlled trial of nicotine chewing-gum. *Br Med J* 1982;285:537–540.

Jenkins AC, Dreslinski GR, Tadros SS, et al: Captopril in hypertension: seven years later. *J Cardiovasc Pharmacol* 1985;7:S96–S101.

Johansson BW: Effect of beta blockade on ventricular fibrillation- and ventricular tachycardia-induced circulatory arrest in acute myocardial infarction. *Am J Cardiol* 1986;57:34F–37F.

Johnston CI: Treatment of hypertension with angiotensin converting enzyme inhibitors. *Aust NZ J Med* 1984;14:509–513.

The Joint National Committee on Detection, Evaluation, and Treatment of High Blood Pressure: A cooperative study. *JAMA* 1977;237:255–261.

The Joint National Committee on Detection, Evaluation, and Treatment of High Blood Pressure: The 1980 report of the Joint National Committee on Detection, Evaluation, and Treatment of High Blood Pressure. *Arch Intern Med* 1980;140:1280–1285.

The Joint National Committee on Detection, Evaluation, and Treatment of High Blood Pressure: The 1984 report of the Joint National Committee on Detection, Evaluation, and Treatment of High Blood Pressure. *Arch Intern Med* 1984;144:1045–1057.

Julius M, Harburg E, Cottington EM, et al: Anger-coping types, blood pressure, and all-cause mortality: a follow-up in Tecumseh, Michigan (1971–1983). *Am J Epidemiol* 1986;124:220–233.

Julius S: The psychophysiology of borderline hypertension, in Weiner H, Hofer MA,

Stunkard AJ (eds): *Brain, Behavior and Bodily Disease.* New York, Raven Press, 1981, pp 293–305.

Kaijser L, Lassers BW, Wahiqvist ML, et al: Myocardial lipid and carbohydrate metabolism in fasting men during prolonged exercise. *J Appl Physiol* 1972;32:847–858.

Kaiser P, Tesch P, Frisk-Holmberg M, et al: Effect of β_1-selective and nonselective β-blockade on work capacity and muscle metabolism. *Clin Physiol* 1986;6:197–207.

Kaneko Y, Yamada K, Ikeda M, et al: Antihypertensive effect of low dose captopril in mild to moderate essential hypertension. *Abstracts of the Internatl Soc Hypertension* 1982;211.

Kannel WB: An overview of the risk factors for cardiovascular disease (chapter 1), in Kaplan NM, Stamler J (eds): *Prevention of Coronary Heart Disease.* Philadelphia, WB Saunders Co, 1983, pp 1–19.

Kannel WB, Abbott RD: A prognostic comparison of asymptomatic left ventricular hypertrophy and unrecognized myocardial infarction: the Framingham study. *Am Heart J* 1986;111:391–397.

Kannel WB, Gordon T, Offut O: Left ventricular hypertrophy by electrocardiogram. Prevalence, incidence and mortality in the Framingham study. *Ann Intern Med* 1969;71:89–105.

Kannel WB, Sorlie P, Gordon T: Labile hypertension: a faulty concept? *Circulation* 1980;61:1183–1187.

Kaplan NM: Whom to treat: the dilemma of mild hypertension. *Am J Heart* 1982;101:867–870.

Kaplan NM: Therapy for mild hypertension: toward a more balanced view. *JAMA* 1983a; 249:365–367.

Kaplan NM: Diabetes and glucose intolerance (chapter 9), in Kaplan NM, Stamler J (eds): *Prevention of Coronary Heart Disease.* Philadelphia, WB Saunders Co, 1983b, pp 113–119.

Kaplan NM: Effects of guanabenz on plasma lipid levels in hypertensive patients. *J Cardiovasc Pharmacol* 1984;6:S841–S846.

Kaplan NM: *Clinical Hypertension* (4th ed). Baltimore, William and Wilkins Co, 1986a, p 186.

Kaplan NM: Treatment of hypertension: drug therapy (chapter 6), in Kaplan NM (ed): *Clinical Hypertension* (4th ed). Baltimore, Williams and Wilkins Co, 1986b, pp 180–272.

Kaplan N, Lieberman E: The therapy of hypertension, in Kaplan N, Lieberman E (eds): *Clinical Hypertension.* Baltimore, Williams and Wilkins Co., 1982, pp 98–192.

Kaplan NM, Meese RB: The calcium deficiency hypothesis of hypertension: a critique. *Ann Intern Med* 1986;105:947–955.

Kaplan RM, Bush JW, Berry CC: Health status index. Category rating versus magnitude estimation for measuring levels of well-being. *Med Care* 1979;17:501–525.

Karatzas P, Clouva P: Effect of methyldopa on cardiac contractility in hypertensive patients, in Zanchetti A (ed): *Aldomet in Worldwide Clinical Experience.* Westpoint, PA, Merck, Sharp & Dohme, 1979, pp 74–83.

Katz S, Akpom CA: A measure of primary sociobiological functions. *Int J Health Serv* 1976;6:493–507.

Katz WA: Compliance. *Seminars Arthritis Rheum* 1982;12(suppl 1):132–135.

Keane WF, Raij L: Relationships among altered glomerular barrier permselectivity, angiotensin II, and mesangial uptake of macromolecules. *Lab Invest* 1985;52:599–604.

Klatsky AL: The relationship of alcohol and the cardiovascular system. *Ann Rev Nutr* 1982;2:51–71.

Klatsky AL, Armstrong MA, Friedman GD: Relations of alcoholic beverage use to subsequent coronary artery disease hospitalization. *Am J Cardiol* 1986a;58:710–714.

Klatsky AL, Friedman GD, Armstrong MA: The relationships between alcoholic beverage use and other traits to blood pressure: a new Kaiser Permanente study. *Circulation* 1986b; 73:628–636.

Klein W, Bradt D, Vrecko K, et al: Role of calcium antagonists in the treatment of essential hypertension. *Circ Res* 1983;52(suppl 1):174–180.

Knowler WC, Bennett PH, Ballintine EJ: Increased incidence of retinopathy in diabetics with elevated blood pressure. A six-year follow-up in Pima Indians. *N Engl J Med* 1980;302:645–650.

Knowles HC: Magnitude of the renal failure problem in diabetic patients. *Kidney Int* 1974;6(suppl 1):S2–S7.

Koch-Weser J: Vasodilator drugs in the treatment of hypertension. *Arch Intern Med* 1974;133:1017–1027.

Kohner EM, Dollery CT, Lowy C, et al: Effect of diuretic therapy on glucose tolerance in hypertensive patients. *Lancet* 1971;1:986–990.

Kokubu T, Itoh I, Kurita H, et al: Effect of prazosin on serum lipids. *J Cardiovasc Pharmacol* 1982;4(suppl 2):S228–S232.

Koshy MC, Mickley D, Bourgiognie J, et al: Physiologic evaluation of a new antihypertensive agent, prazosin HCl. *Circulation* 1977;55:533–537.

Kostis JB, DeFelice EA: The hemodynamic effects of pindolol. *Curr Ther Res* 1983;33: 494–511.

Kramsch DM, Aspen AJ, Abramowitz BM, et al: Reduction of coronary atherosclerosis by moderate conditioning exercise in monkeys on an atherogenic diet. *N Engl J Med* 1981;305:1483–1489.

Krolewski AS, Canessa M, Rand LI, et al: Genetic predisposition to hypertension as a major determinant of development of diabetic nephropathy (abstract). *Kidney Int* 1987;31:388.

Kung M, White JR, Burki NK: The effect of subcutaneously administered terbutaline on serum potassium in asymptomatic adult asthmatics. *Am Rev Resp Dis* 1984;129:329–332.

Kurlen VA, Oliver MF: A metabolic cause for arrhythmias during acute myocardial infarction. *Lancet* 1970;1:813–815.

Kutner B, Fanshel D, Togo AM: *Five Hundred Over Sixty: A Community Survey on Aging.* New York, Russel Sage Foundation, 1956.

Laragh JH: Hormones with the pathogenesis of congestive heart failure: vasopressin, aldosterone, and angiotensin II. *Circulation* 1962;25:1015–1023.

Laragh JH: Mild hypertension: a second opinion on the HDFP Trial. *Drug Ther* 1982;12: 68–74.

Lau K, Eby B: The role of calcium in genetic hypertension. *Hypertension* 1985;7:657–667.

Lawrence DS, Sahay JN, Chatterjee SS, et al: Asthma and beta-blockers. *Eur J Clin Pharmacol* 1982;22:501–509.

Lawton MP: The dimension of morale, in Kent D, Kastenbaum R, Sherwood S (eds):

Research, Planning and Action for the Elderly. New York, Behavioral Publications, 1972, pp 144–165.

Layton CR: Management of hypertension in patients with obstructive airway disease. *J Cardiovasc Med* 1981;(special suppl):43–48.

LeClercq-Meyers, Herchnelz A, Valverde I, et al: Mode of action of clonidine upon islet function. *Diabetes* 1980;29:193–200.

Leibel RL, Hirsch J: Metabolic characterization of obesity. *Ann Intern Med* 1985;103: 1000–1002.

Leitch AG, Hopkin JM, Ellis DA, et al: Failure of propranolol and metoprolol to alter vasodilatory responses to carbon dioxide and exercise. *Br J Clin Pharmacol* 1980;9:493–498.

Leren P, Helgeland A, Holme I: Effect of propranolol and prazosin on serum lipids. The Oslo Study. *Lancet* 1980;2:4–6.

Lerner DJ, Kannel WB: Patterns of coronary heart disease morbidity and mortality in the sexes: a 26-year follow-up of the Framingham population. *Am Heart J* 1986;111:383–390.

Levenson J, Simon AC, Moyse D, et al: Peripheral hemodynamic effects of short-term nadolol administration in essential hypertension. *Am Heart J* 1984;108:1177–1182.

Levine S, Croog SH: What constitutes quality of life? A conceptualization of the dimensions of life quality in healthy populations and patients with cardiovascular disease (chapter 2), in Wenger NK, Mattson ME, Furberg CD, et al (eds): *Assessment of Quality of Life in Clinical Trials of Cardiovascular Therapies.* New York, Le Jacq Publishing Inc, 1984, pp 46–66.

Lewis JG: Adverse reactions to calcium antagonists. *Drugs* 1983;25:196–222.

Lichtenstein E, Mermelstein RJ: Review of approaches to smoking treatment: behavior modification strategies (chapter 44), in Matarazzo JD, Weiss SM, Herd JA, et al (eds): *Behavioral Health: A Handbook of Health Enhancement and Disease Prevention.* New York, John Wiley & Sons, 1984, pp 695–712.

Light KC: Antihypertensive drugs and behavioral performance, in Elias MF, Streeten DHP (eds): *Hypertension and Cognitive Processes.* Mount Desert, ME, Beech Hill Publishing Co, 1980, p 120.

Light KC, Koepke JP, Obrist PA, et al: Psychological stress induces sodium and fluid retention in men at high risk for hypertension. *Science* 1983;220:429–431.

Light RW, Chetty KG, Stansbury DW: Comparison of the effects of labetalol and hydrochlorothiazide on the ventilatory function of hypertensive patients with mild chronic obstructive pulmonary disease. *Am J Med* 1983;75(suppl 4A):109–114.

Lindholm L: Parental obesity combined with hypertension—an indicator of excess risk of hypertension in offspring. *Acta Med Scand* 1984;216:277–285.

Lipid Research Clinics Program: The Lipid Research Clinics Coronary Primary Prevention Trial Results. I. Reduction in incidence of coronary heart disease. *JAMA* 1984;251:351–364.

Lloyd G: Medicine without signs. *Br Med J* 1983;287:539–542.

Lloyd-Mostyn RM, Oram S: Modification by propranolol of cardiovascular effects of induced hypoglycemia. *Lancet* 1975;1:1213–1215.

Lombardo M, Zaini G, Pastori F, et al: Left ventricular mass and function before and after antihypertensive treatment. *J Hypertens* 1983;1:215–219.

Lombrail P, Thibult N, Di Costanzo P, et al: Influence of arterial hypertension in diabetic retinopathy. *Diabetes Metab* 1983;9:297–302.

Loutzenhiser R, Epstein M: Effects of calcium antagonists on renal hemodynamics. *Am J Physiol* 1985;249:F619–F629.

Lowenthal DT, Kendrick ZV: Drug-exercise interactions. *Annu Rev Pharmacol Toxicol* 1985;25:275–305.

Lowenthal DT, Affrime MB, Falkner B, et al: Potassium disposition and neuroendocrine effects of propranolol, methyldopa and clonidine during dynamic exercise. *Clin Exp Hypertens-Theory Pract* 1982a;A4(9–10):1895–1911.

Lowenthal DT, Affrime MB, Rosenthal L, et al: Dynamic and biochemical responses to single and repeated doses of clonidine during dynamic physical activity. *Clin Pharmacol Ther* 1982b;32:18–24.

Lowenthal DT, Dickerman D, Saris SD, et al: The effect of pharmacological interaction on central and peripheral alpha-receptors and pressor response to static exercise. *Ann Sports Med* 1984a;1(3):100–104.

Lowenthal DT, Saris SD, Packer J, et al: The mechanisms of action and the clinical pharmacology of beta adrenergic blocking drugs. *Am J Med* 1984b;77(suppl 4A):119–127.

Luft FC, Weinberger MH, Grim CE, et al: Sodium sensitivity in normotensive human subjects. *Ann Intern Med* 1983;98:758–762.

Lund-Johansen P: Hemodynamics in early essential hypertension. *Acta Med Scand* 1967; 181(suppl 482):1–101.

Lund-Johansen P: Hemodynamic changes in long-term diuretic therapy of essential hypertension. A comparative study of chlorthalidone, polythiazide and hydrochlorothiazide. *Acta Med Scand* 1970;187:509–518.

Lund-Johansen P: Hemodynamic changes in long-term alpha methyldopa therapy of essential hypertension. *Acta Med Scand* 1972;192:221–226.

Lund-Johansen P: Hemodynamic changes at rest and during exercise in long-term clonidine therapy of essential hypertension. *Acta Med Scand* 1974;195:111–117.

Lund-Johansen P: Hemodynamic changes at rest and during exercise in long-term prazosin therapy for essential hypertension, in *Postgrad Med Symp Prazosin*. New York, McGraw-Hill, 1975, p 45.

Lund-Johansen P: Hemodynamic long-term effects of timolol at rest and during exercise in essential hypertension. *Acta Med Scand* 1976;199:263–267.

Lund-Johansen P: Alpha-methyldopa and beta-blockers in hypertension—a comparison of their hemodynamic effects. *Clin Exp Pharmacol Physiol* 1978a;4(suppl):23–34.

Lund-Johansen P: Spontaneous changes in central hemodynamics in essential hypertension—a 10 year follow-up study, in Onesti G, Klimt F (eds): *Hypertension: Determinants, Complications and Intervention*. New York, Grune and Stratton, 1978b, pp 201–209.

Lund-Johansen P: Hemodynamics in essential hypertension. *Clin Sci* 1980;59:343S–354S.

Lund-Johansen P: Hemodynamic effects of verapamil in essential hypertension at rest and during exercise. *Acta Med Scand* 1984;(suppl 681):109–116.

Lundborg P, Astrom H, Bengtsson C, et al: Effect of beta-adrenoceptor blockade on exercise performance and metabolism. *Clin Sci* 1981;61:299–305.

MacDougall JM, Dembroski TM, Slaats S, et al: Selective cardiovascular effects of stress and cigarette smoking. *J Hum Stress* 1983;9:13–21.

Mace PJE, Littler WA, Glover DR, et al: Regression of left ventricular hypertrophy in hypertension: comparative effects of three different drugs. *J Cardiovasc Pharmacol* 1985;7: S52–S55.

MacGregor GA: Sodium is more important than calcium in essential hypertension. *Hypertension* 1985;7:628–637.

MacMahon SW, Macdonald GJ: Antihypertensive treatment and plasma lipoprotein levels: the association in data from a population study. *Am J Med* 1986;80(suppl 2A):40–47.

MacMahon SW, Norton RN: Alcohol and hypertension: implications for prevention and treatment. *Ann Intern Med* 1986;105:124–125.

Malini PL, Strocchi E, Ambrosini E: Comparison of the effects of timolol and propranolol on renal hemodynamics. *NZ Med J* 1983;96:892–893.

Manhem P, Bramnert M, Hulthen UL, et al: The effect of captopril on catecholamines, renin activity, angiotensin II and aldosterone in plasma during physical exercise in hypertensive patients. *Eur J Clin Invest* 1981;11:389–395.

Manuck SB, Kaplan SR, Clarkson TB: Behavioral-induced heart rate reactivity and atherosclerosis in cynomolgus monkeys. *Psychosom Med* 1983;45:95–108.

Massie BM, Hirsch AT, Inouye IK, et al: Calcium channel blockers as antihypertensive agents. *Am J Med* 1984;77(4A):135–142.

Materson BJ: Monotherapy of hypertension with angiotensin-converting enzyme inhibitors. *Am J Med* 1984;77(4A):128–134.

Materson BJ: Sexual dysfunction during antihypertensive treatment. *Prog in Pharmacol* 1985a;6:117–124.

Materson BJ: Diuretic-associated hypokalemia (editorial). *Arch Intern Med* 1985b;145: 1966–1967.

Materson BJ: Hypertension and concomitant disease: guidelines for treatment. *Drug Therapy* 1985c;15:177–188.

Materson BJ: Thiazides increase cardiovascular risk. *Drug Therapy* 1986a;16:51–55.

Materson BJ: Adverse effects of antihypertensive treatment. *Cardiol Clinics* 1986b;4: 105–115.

Mauer SM, Steffes MW, Azar S, et al: The effects of Goldblatt hypertension on development of the glomerular lesions of diabetes mellitus in the rat. *Diabetes* 1978;27:738–744.

Mauer S, Steffes MW, Sutherland D, et al: Studies of the rate of regression of the glomerular lesions in diabetic rats treated with pancreatic islet transplantation. *Diabetes* 1974;24: 280–285.

Maxwell MH, Kushiro T, Dornfeld LP, et al: Blood pressure changes in obese hypertensive subjects during rapid weight loss: comparison of restricted *vs* unchanged salt intake. *Arch Intern Med* 1984;144:1581–1584.

McCarron DA: Is calcium more important than sodium in the pathogenesis of essential hypertension? *Hypertension* 1985;7:607–627.

McHenry PL, Faris JV, Jordari JW, et al: Comparative study of cardiovascular function and ventricular premature complexes in smokers and nonsmokers during maximal treadmill exercise. *Am J Cardiol* 1977;39:493–498.

McKenna WJ, Borggefe M, England D, et al: The natural history of left ventricular hypertrophy in hypertrophic cardiomyopathy: an electrocardiographic study. *Circulation* 1982;66:1233–1240.

McKinney ME, Miner MH, Ruddel H, et al: The standardized mental stress test protocol: test-retest reliability and comparison with ambulatory blood pressure monitoring. *Psychophysiol* 1985;22:453–463.

McNamara JJ, Molot MA, Stremple JF, et al: Coronary artery disease in combat casualties in Vietnam. *JAMA* 1971;216:1185–1187.

McNeir DM, Lorr M, Droppleman LF: *Profile of Mood States*. San Diego, Educational and Industrial Testing Service, 1971.

Meade TW, Brozovic M, Chakrabarti RR, et al: Haemostatic function and ischaemic heart disease: principal results of the Northwick Park heart study. *Lancet* 1986;2:533–537.

Medical Research Council Working Party: MRC trial of treatment of mild hypertension: principal results. *Br Med J* 1985;291:97–104.

Medical Research Council Working Party on Mild to Moderate Hypertension: Adverse reactions to bendrofluazide and propranolol for the treatment of mild hypertension. *Lancet* 1981:2:539–543.

Meenan RF, Gertman PM, Masen JH: Measuring health status in arthritis: the arthritis impact measurement scales. *Arthritis Rheum* 1980;23:146–152.

Messerli FH: Cardiovascular adaptations to obesity and arterial hypertension: detrimental or beneficial? *Int J Cardiol* 1983;3:94–97.

Messerli FH, Ventura HO, Amodeo C: Osler's maneuver and pseudohypertension. *N Engl J Med* 1985;312:1348–1351.

Messerli FH, Dreslinski GR, Husserl FE, et al: Antiadrenergic therapy: special aspects in hypertension in the elderly. *Hypertension* 1981a;3(suppl 2):2–12.

Messerli FH, Frohlich ED, Suarez DH, et al: Borderline hypertension: relationship between age, hemodynamics, circulating catecholamines. *Circulation* 1981b;64:760–764.

Messerli FH, Ventura HO, Elizardi DJ, et al: Hypertension and sudden death: increased ventricular ectopic activity in left ventricular hypertrophy. *Am J Med* 1984;77:18–22.

Metz SA, Halter JB, Robertson RP: Induction of defective insulin secretion of long-term efficacy and safety of labetalol in treatment of hypertension. *Am J Med* 1983;75(suppl 4A):54–67.

Michelson EL, Frishman WH, Lewis JH, et al: Multicenter clinical evaluation of long-term efficacy and safety of labetalol in treatment of hypertension. *Am J Med* 1983;75(suppl 4A):68–80.

Mitas JA, Levy SB, Holle R, et al: Urinary kallikrein activity in the hypertension of renal parenchymal disease. *N Eng J Med* 1978;299:162–165.

Mitchell HC, Graham RM, Pettinger WA: Renal function during long-term treatment of hypertension with minoxidil. Comparison of benign and malignant hypertension. *Ann Intern Med* 1980;93:676–681.

Miyazaki S, Miura K, Kasai Y, et al: Relief from digital vasospasm by treatment with captopril and its complete inhibition by serine proteinase inhibitors in Raynaud's phenomenon. *Br Med J* 1982;284:310–311.

Modan M, Halhin H, Almog S, et al: Hyperinsulinemia: a link between hypertension, obesity and glucose intolerance. *J Clin Invest* 1985;75:809–817.

Mogensen CE: Progression of nephropathy in long-term diabetics with proteinuria and effect of initial antihypertensive treatment. *Scan J Clin Lab Invest* 1976a;36:383–388.

Mogensen CE: Renal function changes in diabetes. *Diabetes* 1976b;25:872–879.

Mogensen CE: Long term antihypertensive therapy reduces the rate of decline in kidney function in diabetic nephropathy. *Lancet* 1983;1:1175.

Mogensen CE: Microalbuminuria as a predictor of clinical diabetic nephropathy. *Kidney Int* 1987;31:673–689.

Mogensen CE, Christensen CK: Predicting diabetic nephropathy in insulin dependent patients. *N Eng J Med* 1984;311:89–93.

Mooney AJ II: Alcohol use (chapter 10), in Taylor RB, Ureda JR, Denham JW (eds): *Health Promotion: Principles and Clinical Applications.* Norwalk, CT, Appleton-Century-Crofts, 1982, pp 233–258.

Moore RD, Pearson TA: Moderate alcohol consumption and coronary artery disease: a review. *Medicine* 1986;65:242–267.

Morganroth J: Premature ventricular complexes: diagnosis and indications for therapy. *JAMA* 1984;252:673–676.

Morin Y, Turmel L, Fortier J: Methyldopa: clinical studies in arterial hypertension. *Am J Med Sci* 1964;248:633–639.

Moser M: "Less severe" hypertension: should it be treated? *Am Heart J* 1982;101:465–472.

Moser M: Historical perspective on the management of hypertension. *Am J Med* 1986; 80(suppl 5B):1–11.

Moskowitz RM, Piccini PA, Nacarelli GV, et al: Nifedipine therapy for stable angina pectoris: preliminary results of effects on angina frequency and treadmill exercise response. *Am J Cardiol* 1979;44:811–816.

Moss AJ: Blood pressure in children with diabetes mellitus. *Pediatrics* 1962;30:932–936.

Moyer JH: Hydralazine (apresoline) hydrochloride. Pharmacological observations and clinical results in the therapy of hypertension. *Arch Intern Med* 1953;91:419–439.

Mujais SK, Fouad FM, Tarazi RC: Reversal of left ventricular hypertrophy with captopril: heterogeneity of response among hypertensive patients. *Clin Cardiol* 1983;6:595–602.

Multiple Risk Factor Intervention Trial Research Group: Multiple risk factor intervention trial: risk factor changes in mortality results. *JAMA* 1982;248:1465–1477.

Multiple Risk Factor Intervention Trial Research Group: Baseline rest electrocardiographic abnormalities, antihypertensive treatment, and mortality in the multiple risk factor intervention trial. *Am J Cardiol* 1985;55:1–15.

Murphy MH, Kohner E, Lewis PJ, et al: Glucose intolerance in hypertensive patients treated with diuretics: a fourteen-year follow-up. *Lancet* 1982;2:1293–1295.

Najman JM, Levine S: Evaluating the impact of medical care and technologies on the quality of life: a review and critique. *Soc Sci Med* 1981;15F:107–115.

Nelson GIC, Donnelly GL, Hunyor SN: Hemodynamic effects of sustained treatment with prazosin and metoprolol, alone and in combination, in borderline hypertensive heart failure. *J Cardiovasc Pharmacol* 1982;4:240–245.

Neugarten BL, Havighurst RJ, Tobin SS: Measurement of life satisfaction. *J Gerontol* 1961;16:134–143.

Newman WP III, Freedman DS, Voors AW, et al: Relation of serum lipoprotein levels and systolic blood pressure to early atherosclerosis, the Bogalusa heart study. *N Engl J Med* 1986;314:138–144.

Newsholme EA: The regulation of intracellular and extracellular fuel supply during sustained exercise. *Ann NY Acad Sci* 1977;30:81–89.

Nicholls MG, Espiner EA, Ikram H, et al: Angiotensin II is more potent than potassium in regulating aldosterone in cardiac failure: evidence during captopril therapy. *J Clin Endo Metab* 1981;52:1253–1256.

Nicholson JP, Alderman MH, Pickering TG, et al: Cigarette smoking and renovascular hypertension. *Lancet* 1983;ii:765–766.

Nies AS: Adverse reactions and interactions limiting the use of antihypertensive drugs. *Am J Med* 1975;58:495–503.

Nordrehaug JE, von der Lippe G: Hypokalaemia and ventricular fibrillation in acute myocardial infarction. *Br Heart J* 1983;50:525–529.

Oberfield SE, Case DB, Levine LS, et al: Use of the oral angiotensin I-converting enzyme inhibitor (captopril) in childhood malignant hypertension. *J Pedriatr* 1979;95:641-644.

O'Connor DT, Preston RA, Sasso EH: Renal perfusion changes during treatment of essential hypertension: prazosin versus propranolol. *J Cardiovasc Pharmacol* 1978;1(suppl): S38–S42.

Ogilvie RI: Cardiovascular response to exercise under increasing doses of chlorthalidone. *Eur J Clin Pharmacol* 1976;9:339–344.

Olshan AR, O'Connor DT, Cohen IM, et al: Hypertension in adult onset diabetes mellitus: abnormal renal hemodynamics and endogenous vasoregulatory factors. *Am J Kidney Dis* 1982;2:271–280.

O'Malley K, O'Callaghan WG, Laher MS, et al: β-Adrenoceptor blocking drugs and renal blood flow with special reference to the elderly. *Drugs* 1983;25(suppl 2):103–107.

Onesti G: Antihypertensives and their modes of action. *Drug Ther* 1978;8:35–48.

Ople LH: Metabolism of free fatty acids, glucose and catecholamines in acute myocardial infarction. Relation to myocardial ischemia and infarct size. *Am J Cardiol* 1975;36:938–953.

O'Rourke MF: Arterial function in health and disease. Edinburgh, Churchill Livingstone, 1982, pp 196–252.

O'Rourke RA: Rationale for calcium entry-blocking drugs in systemic hypertension complicated by coronary artery disease. *Am J Cardiol* 1985;56:34H–40H.

Oster JR, Materson BJ: Pseudohypertension: a diagnostic dilemma. *J Clin Hypertension* 1986;2:307–313.

Ostman J, Arner P, Maglund K, et al: Effect of metoprolol and alprenolol on the metabolic, hormonal, and hemodynamic response to insulin-induced hypoglycemia in hypertensive, insulin dependent diabetics. *Acta Med Scand* 1982;211:381–385.

Packer M, Lee WH, Yushak M, et al: Comparison of captopril and enalapril in patients with severe chronic heart failure. *N Engl J Med* 1986;315:847–853.

Pacy PJ, Dodson P, Kubicki AJ, et al: Comparison of the hypotensive and metabolic effects of bendrogluazide therapy and a high fibre, low fat, low sodium diet in diabetic subjects with mild hypertension. *J Hypertens* 1984;2:215–220.

Paffenbarger RS Jr, Hyde RT, Wing AL, et al: Physical activity, all-cause mortality, and longevity of college alumni. *N Engl J Med* 1986;314:605–613.

Pagani F, Fiorella G, Benco R, et al: Comparison of the effects of short-term treatment with guanfacine and clonidine on glucose metabolism, plasma renin activity and some anterior pituitary hormones. *Curr Ther Res* 1984;36:155–162.

Palmer GI, Ziegler MG, Lake CR: Response of norepinephrine and blood pressure to stress increases with age. *J Gerentol* 1978;33:482–485.

Panidis IP, Kotler MN, Ren JF, et al: Development and regression of left ventricular hypertrophy. *J Am Coll Cardiol* 1984;3:1309–1320.

Parijs J, Joossens JV, Van der Linden L, et al: Moderate sodium restriction and diuretics in the treatment of hypertension. *Am Heart J* 1973;85:22–34.

Parving HH, Andersen AR, Smidt UM, et al: Diabetic nephropathy and arterial hypertension. *Diabetologia* 1983a;24:10–12.

Parving HH, Smidt UM, Andersen AR, et al: Early aggressive antihypertensive therapy reduces the rate of decline in kidney function in diabetic nephropathy. *Lancet* 1983b;1:1175–1178.

Parving HH, Smidt UM, Friisberg B, et al: A prospective study of glomerular filtration rate and arterial blood pressure in insulin dependent diabetics with diabetic nephropathy. *Diabetologia* 1981;20:457–461.

Pasanisi F, Ferrara AL, Iovine C, et al: Effects of nifedipine on insulin secretion and plasma lipids in hypertensive patients. *Curr Ther Res* 1986;39:894–899.

Pasotti C, Capra A, Fiorello G, et al: Effects of pindolol and metoprolol on plasma lipids and lipoproteins. *Br J Clin Pharmacol* 1982;13(suppl 2):435S–439S.

Pearlman RA, Jansen A: The use of quality-of-life considerations in medical decision making. *J Am Geriatr Soc* 1985;33:344–352.

Pell S, D'Alanza CA: Some aspects of hypertension in diabetes mellitus. *JAMA* 1967;202:104.

Perry HM (chairman): Recommendations for a National High Blood Pressure Program Data Base for Effective Antihypertensive Therapy, Report of Task Force I, DHEW publication No (NIH) 75-593. Bethesda, MD, US Dept of Health, Education, and Welfare, 1973.

Perry HM Jr: Some wrong-way chemical changes during antihypertensive treatment: comparison of indapamide and related agents. *Am Heart J* 1983;106:251–257.

Pershadsingh HA, Grant N: Association of diltiazem therapy with increased insulin resistance in a patient with type I diabetes mellitus. *JAMA* 1987;257:930–931.

Pettinger WA, Keeton K: Altered renin release and propranolol potentiation of vasodilatory drug hypotension. *J Clin Invest* 1959;55:236–240.

Pfeffer JM, Pfeffer MA, Braunwald E: Influence of chronic captopril therapy on the infarcted left ventricle of the rat. *Circulation Res* 1985a;57:84–95.

Pfeffer MA, Pfeffer JM, Steinberg C, et al: Survival after an experimental myocardial infarction: beneficial effects of long-term therapy with captopril. *Circulation* 1985b;72:406–412.

Phillipson BE, Rothrock DW, Connor WE, et al: Reduction of plasma lipids, lipoproteins, and apoproteins by dietary fish oils in patients with hypertriglyceridemia. *N Engl J Med* 1985;312:1210–1216.

Pickering TG, Base DB, Sullivan PA, et al: Comparison of antihypertensive and hormonal effects of captopril and propranolol at rest and during exercise. *Am J Cardiol* 1982;49:1566–1568.

Pickup J, Sherwin RS, Tamborlance WV, et al: The Kroc Collaborative Study Group. The pump life: patient responses and clinical and technical problems. *Diabetes* 1985;34(suppl 3):37–41.

Pierpont G, Cohn JN: Comparison of the renal effects of vasodilators used to treat congestive heart failure. *Cardiovasc Rev Rep* 1981;2:1199–1209.

Plough AL, Salem SR, Shwartz M, et al: Case mix in end-stage renal disease: differences between patients in hospital-based and free-standing treatment facilities. *N Engl J Med* 1984;310:1432–1436.

Pratt CM, Welton DE, Squires WG Jr, et al: Demonstration of training effect during chronic beta-adrenergic blockade in patients with coronary artery disease. *Circulation* 1981;64:1125–1129.

Preston RA, O'Connor DT, Stone RA: Prazosin and renal hemodynamics: arterial vasodilation during therapy of essential hypertension in man. *J Cardiovasc Pharmacol* 1979;1:277–286.

Raij L: Role of hypertension in progressive glomerular injury in glomerulonephritis. *Hypertension* 1986;8(suppl 1):130–133.

Raij L, Chiou X, Oldens R, et al: Therapeutic implications of hypertension-induced glomerular injury. Comparison of enalapril and a combination of hydralazine, reserpine and hydrochlorothiazide in an experimental model. *Am J Med* 1985;79(suppl 3C):37–41.

Raij L, Keane WF: Glomerular mesangium: its function and relationship to angiotensin II. *Am J Med* 1985;79 (suppl 3C):24–30.

Ram CVS, Anderson RJ, Hart GR, et al: Alpha adrenergic blockage by prazosin in therapy of essential hypertension. *Clin Pharmacol Ther* 1981;29:719–722.

Rapaport MI, Heard HF: Thiazide-induced glucose intolerance treated with potassium. *Arch Intern Med* 1964;113:405–408.

Rasmussen HS, Aurup P, Hojberg S, et al: Magnesium and acute myocardial infarction. *Arch Intern Med* 1986a;146:872–874.

Rasmussen HS, Norregard P, Lindeneg O, et al: Intravenous magnesium in acute myocardial infarction. *Lancet* 1986b;1:234–235.

Regan TJ: Alcoholic cardiomyopathy. *Prog Cardiovasc Dis* 1984;27:141–152.

Reid JL, White KF, Struthers AD: Epinephrine-induced hypokalemia: the role of beta adrenoceptors. *Am J Cardiol* 1986;57:23F–27F.

Reidenberg MM, Lowenthal DT: Adverse non-drug reactions. *N Engl J Med* 1968;279:678–679.

Report by the Management Committee: The Australian therapeutic trial in mild hypertension. *Lancet* 1980;1:1261–1267.

Rett K, Jarach KW, Wicklmayr M: Angiotensin-converting enzyme inhibition in diabetes: experimental and human experience. *Postgrad Med J* 1986;62(suppl 1):59–64.

Riendl A, Gotshall RW, Reinke JA, et al: Cardiovascular response of human subjects to isometric contraction of large and small muscle groups. *Proc Soc Exp Biol Med* 1977;154:171–174.

Robertson JIS: The treatment of hypertension and quality of life. *J Hypertens* 1985;3(suppl 2):S89–S90.

Rodin J, Wack JT: The relationship between cigarette smoking and body weight: a health promotion dilemma? (chapter 42), in Matarazzo JD, Weiss SM, Herd JA, et al (eds): *Behavioral Health: A Handbook of Health Enhancement and Disease Prevention*. New York, John Wiley & Sons, 1984, pp 671–690.

Roe JW, Tobin JD, Rose RM, et al: Effects of experimental potassium deficiency on glucose and insulin metabolism. *Metabolism* 1980;29:498–502.

Roehmoldt ME, Paumbo PH, Qhisnant JP, et al: Transient ischemic attack and stroke in a community-based diabetic cohort. *Mayo Clinic Proc* 1983;58:56–58.

Romero JC, Raij L, Granger JP, et al: Multiple effects of calcium entry blockers on renal function in hypertension. *Hypertension* 1987;10:140–151.

Roos JC, Boer P, Loomons HA, et al: Haemodynamic and hormonal changes during acute and chronic diuretic treatment in essential hypertension. *Eur J Clin Pharmacol* 1981;19:107–112.

Rose G, Shipley M: Plasma cholesterol concentration and death from coronary heart disease: 10 year results of the Whitehall study. *Br Med J* 1986;293:306–307.

Rosenthal L, Affrime MB, Lowenthal DT, et al: Biochemical and dynamic responses to single and repeated doses of methyldopa and propranolol during dynamic physical activity. *Clin Pharmacol Ther* 1982;32:701–710.

Rouleau JL, Chatterjee K, Benge W, et al: Alterations in left ventricular function and coronary hemodynamics with captopril, hydralazine and prazosin in chronic ischemic heart failure: a comparative study. *Circulation* 1982;65:671–678.

Rowe JW, Tobin JD, Rosa RM, et al: Effect of experimental protassium deficiency on glucose and insulin metabolism. *Metabolism* 1980;29:489–502.

Ruilope LM, Miranda B, Morales JM, et al: Control of hypertension with a converting enzyme inhibitor slows progression of renal insufficiency in human chronic renal failure (abstract) *Kidney Int* 1987;31:215.

Rystedt LL, Williams GH, Hollenberg NK: The renal and endocrine response to saline infusion in essential hypertension. *Hypertension* 1986;8:217–222.

Sachs FM, Dzau VJ: Adrenergic effects on plasma lipoprotein metabolism. *Am J Med* 1986;80(suppl 2A):71–81.

Sackett DL, Chambers LW, MacPherson AS, et al: The development and applications of indices of health: general method and summary of results. *Am J Public Health* 1977;67:423–428.

Sackett DL, Haynes RB, Gibson ES, et al: Randomized clinical trial of strategies for improving medication compliance in primary hypertension. *Lancet* 1975;1:1205–1207.

Safar ME, London GM, Levenson JA, et al: Effect of alpha-methyldopa on cardiac output in hypertension. *Clin Pharmacol Ther* 1979;25:266–272.

Safar ME, Weiss YA, Levenson JA, et al: Hemodynamic study of 85 patients with borderline hypertension. *Am J Cardiol* 1973;31:315–319.

Salena BJ: Chronic cough and the use of captopril: unmasking asthma (letter). *Arch Intern Med* 1986;146:202–203.

Samuelsson O, Wikstrand J, Wilhelmsen L, et al: Heart and kidney involvement during antihypertensive treatment: results from the primary preventive trial in Göteborg, Sweden. *Acta Med Scan* 1984;215:305–311.

Sannerstedt R, Varnanskes E, Werko L: Hemodynamic effects of methyldopa (Aldomet) at rest and during exercise in patients with arterial hypertension. *Acta Med Scand* 1962;171:75–82.

Sannerstedt R, Wasir H, Henning R, et al: Systemic hemodynamics in mild arterial hypertension before and after physical training. *Clin Sci Mol Med* 1973;45(suppl 1):145–152.

Sassano P, Chatellier G, Alhenc-Gelas F, et al: Antihypertensive effect of enalapril as first step treatment of mild and moderate uncomplicated essential hypertension. *Am J Med* 1984;77(suppl 2A):18–22.

Savage DD, Garrison RJ, Castelli WP: Echocardiographic left ventricular hypertrophy in the general population is associated with increased 2-year mortality, independent of standard coronary risk factors—the Framingham study (abstract). *Abstract 25th Conference on Cardiovascular Epidemiology, March 7–9, 1985: Cardiovascular Disease Epidemiology Newsletter No 37*, American Heart Association, 1985, p 22.

Schatzkin A, Cupples LA, Heeren T, et al: The epidemiology of sudden unexpected death: risk factors for men and women in the Framingham heart study. *Am Heart J* 1984;107:1300–1306.

Schoenfeld MY, Goldberger E: Hypercholesterolemia induced by thiazides: a pilot study. *Curr Ther Res* 1964;6:180–184.

Semple PF, Herd GW: Cough and wheeze caused by inhibitors of angiotensin-converting enzyme (letter). *N Engl J Med* 1986;314:61.

Shah S, Khatri I, Freis ED: Mechanisms of antihypertensive effects of thiazide diuretics. *Am Heart J* 1978;95:611–618.

Shaper AG, Pocock SJ, Phillips AN, et al: Identifying men at high risk of heart attacks: strategy for use in general practice. *Br Med J* 1986;293:474–479.

Shionoiri H, Noda K, Miyamoto K, et al: Glucose tolerance during chronic prazosin therapy in patients with essential hypertension. *Curr Ther Res* 1986;40:171–180.

Shopsin B, Hirsch J, Gershon S: Visual hallucinations and propranolol. *Biol Psychiatry* 1975;10:105–107.

Silke B, Nelson GIC, Ahuja RC, et al: Beta-blockade in ischemic heart disease—influence of concomitant ISA or alpha-blockade on hemodynamic profile. *Postgrad Med* 1983;59(suppl 3):45–52.

Simon AC, Levenson JA, Bouthier J, et al: Effects of acute and chronic angiotensin-converting enzyme inhibition on large arteries in human hypertension. *J Cardiovasc Pharmacol* 1985;7(suppl 1):S45–S51.

Sims EAH: Mechanisms of hypertension in the syndromes of obesity. *Int J Obesity* 1981;5(suppl 1):9–18.

Singleton W, Taylor CR: Effect of trimazosin on serum lipid profiles in hypertensive patients. *Am Heart J* 1983;106:1265–1268.

Siscovick DS, LaPorte RE, Newman JM: The disease-specific benefits and risks of physical activity and exercise. *Public Health Rep* 1985;100:180–188.

Sklar J, Johnston DG, Overlie P, et al: The effects of a cardioselective (metoprolol) and a nonselective (propranolol) beta-adrenergic blocker on the response to dynamic exercise in normal men. *Circulation* 1982;65:894–899.

Smith WM: Treatment of mild hypertension: results of a ten-year intervention trial. US Public Health Service Hospitals Cooperative Study Group. *Circ Res* 1977;40(suppl 1):98–105.

Smith WM: Long-term clinical experience with enalapril, in Doyle AE, Beam AG (eds): *Hypertension and the Angiotensin System: Therapeutic Approaches*. New York, Raven Press, 1984, pp 261–279.

Sotaniemi EA, Anttila M, Rautio A, et al: Propranolol and sotalol metabolism after a drinking party. *Clin Pharmacol Ther* 1981;29:705–710.

Sperduto WA, Thompson HS, O'Brien RM: The effect of target behavior monitoring on weight loss and completion rate in a behavior modification program for weight reduction. *Addict Behav* 1986;11:337–340.

Sperzel WD, Glassman HN, Jordan DC, et al: Overall safety of terazosin as an antihypertensive agent. *Am J Med* 1986;80(suppl 5B):77–81.

Spivack C, Ocken S, Frishman WH: Calcium antagonists clinical use in the treatment of systemic hypertension. *Drugs* 1983;25:154–177.

Stamler J, Wentworth D, Neaton JD: Prevalence and prognostic significance of hypercholesterolemia in men with hypertension: prospective data on the primary screenees of the Multiple Risk Factor Intervention Trial. *Am J Med* 1986;80(suppl 2A):33–36.

Stamler R, Stamler J, Gosch FC, et al: Initial antihypertensive drug therapy: alpha blocker or diuretic. *Am J Med* 1986;80(suppl 2A):90–93.

Steffes WM, Brown D, Mauer SM: Diabetic glomerulopathy following uinlateral nephrectomy in the rat. *Diabetes* 1978;27:35–41.

Stein DT, Lowenthal DT, Porter RS, et al: Effects of nifedipine and verapamil on isometric and dynamic exercise in normal subjects. *Am J Cardiol* 1984;54:386–389.

Steiner JA, Cooper R, McPherson K, et al: Effect of β-adrenergic antagonists on prevalence of peripheral vascular symptoms in hypertensive patients. *Br J Clin Pharmacol* 1982; 14:833–837.

Stene-Larsen G, Ask JA, Helle KB, et al: Activation of cardiac β_2 adrenoceptors in the human heart. *Am J Cardiol* 1986;57:7F–10F.

Stephen SA: Unwanted effects of propranolol. *Am J Cardiol* 1966;18:463–472.

Stern MT: The recent decline in ischemic heart disease mortality. *Ann Intern Med* 1979;91:630–640.

Stevenson JG, Umstead GS: Sexual dysfunction due to antihypertensive agents. *Drug Intell Clin Pharm* 1984;18:113–121.

Stewart DE, Ikram H, Espiner EA, et al: Arrhythmogenic potential of diuretic-induced hypokalemia in patients with mild hypertension and ischaemic heart disease. *Br Heart J* 1985;54:290–297.

Stone MC, Thorpe JM: Plasma fibrinogen – a major coronary risk factor. *J Royal Coll Gen Pract* 1985;35:565–569.

Struthers AD, Murphy MB, Dollery CT: Glucose tolerance during antihypertensive therapy in patients with diabetes mellitus. *Hypertension* 1985;7(suppl II):II95–II101.

Struthers AD, Whitesmith R, Reid JL: Prior thiazide diuretic treatment increases adrenaline-induced hypokalemia. *Lancet* 1983;1:1358–1361.

Subcommittee on Nonpharmacological Therapy of the 1984 Joint National Committee on Detection, Evaluation, and Treatment of High Blood Pressure: Nonpharmacological approaches to the control of high blood pressure. *Hypertension* 1986;8:444–467.

Subramanian B, Bowles MH, Davies AB, et al: Combined therapy with verapamil and propranolol in chronic stable angina. *Am J Cardiol* 1982;49:125–132.

Sugimoto T, Rosansky SJ: The incidence of treated end stage renal disease in the eastern United States: 1973–1979. *Am J Public Health* 1984;74:14–17.

Taguma Y, Kitamoto Y, Futaki G, et al: Effect of captopril on heavy proteinuria in azotemic diabetics. *NEnglJ Med* 1985;313:1617–1620.

Tarazi RC, Dustan HP: Beta-adrenergic blockade in hypertension. Practical and theoretical implications of long-term hemodynamic variations. *Am J Cardiol* 1972;29:633–640.

Tarazi RC, Dustan HP: Hemodynamic effects of propranolol in hypertension. *Postgrad Med J* 1976;52(suppl IV):92–100.

Taylor SH: In Marshall AS, Barritt DW (eds): *The Hypertensive Patient*. Kent, England, Pitman Medical Press, 1980.

Taylor RB, Denham JW, Ureda JR: Health promotion: a perspective (chapter 1), in Taylor RB, Ureda JR, Denham JW (eds): *Health Promotion: Principles and Clinical Applications*. Norwalk, CT, Appleton-Century-Crofts, 1982, pp 1–18.

Temmar MM, Safar ME, Levenson JA, et al: Regional blood flow in borderline and sustained essential hypertension. *Clin Sci* 1981;60:653–658.

Terry LL: After 20 years of antismoking effort, where do we stand? *Consultant* 1984;Feb;307–315.

Tesch PA, Kaiser P: Effects of beta adrenergic blockade on O_2 uptake during submaximal and maximal exercise. *J Appl Physiol* 1983;54:901–905.

Testa MA: Quality of life during antihypertensive therapy: techniques for clinical assessment and evaluation. *Br J Clin Pharmacol* 1987a;23:9S–13S.

Testa MA: Interpreting quality-of-life clinical trial data for use in the clinical practice of antihypertensive therapy. *J Hypertens* 1987b;5(suppl 1):S9–S13.

Thurm RH, Alexander JC: Captopril in the treatment of scleroderma renal crisis. *Arch Intern Med* 1984;144:7833–7835.

Tobian L: Hypertension and obesity. *N Eng J Med* 1978;298:46–48.

Tobian L: Human essential hypertension: implications of animal studies. *Ann Intern Med* 1983;98(part 2):729–734.

Touvonen S, Mustala O: Diabetogenic action of furosemide. *Br Med J* 1966;1:920–921.

Trost BN, Weidman P, Beretta-Piccoli C: Antihypertensive therapy in diabetic patients. *Hypertension* 1985;7:102–108.

Tsukiyama H, Otsuka K, Higuma K: Effects of beta-adrenoceptor antagonists on central hemodynamics in essential hypertension. *Br J Clin Pharmacol* 1982;13(suppl):269S–278S.

Tuomilehto J, Nissinen A, Salonen J, et al: Long term effects of cessation of smoking on body weight, blood pressure, and serum cholesterol in the middle-aged population with high blood pressure. *Addict Behav* 1986;11:1–9.

Turner RC: United Kingdom Prospective Diabetes Survey II. Prevalence of hypertension and hypotensive therapy in patients with newly diagnosed diabetes. *Hypertension* 1985;7:118–123.

US Bureau of the Census: Statistical Abstract of the United States: 1986 (106th ed). Washington, DC, 1985, p 985.

US Public Health Service: *Smoking and Health: A Report of the Surgeon General*. DHEW (PHS) Publ No 79-50066, US Dept of Health, Education and Welfare, Public Health Service, 1979.

Vaillant GE: Natural history of male psychologic health: effects of mental health on physical health. *N Engl J Med* 1979;23:1249–1254.

Vale JA, Jeffreys DB: Peripheral gangrene complicating beta blockade (letter). *Lancet* 1978;1:1216.

Veit CT, Ware JE: The structure of psychological distress and well-being in general populations. *J Consult Clin Psychol* 1983;51:730–742.

Velasco M, Silva H, Morilla J, et al: Effect of prazosin on blood lipids and on thyroid function in hypertensive patients. *J Cardiovasc Pharmacol* 1982;4(suppl 2):S225–S227.

Ventura HO, Frohlich ED, Messerli FH, et al: Cardiovascular effects and regional blood flow distribution associated with angiotensin converting enzyme inhibition (captopril) in essential hypertension. *Am J Cardiol* 1985;55:1023–1026.

Veterans Administration Cooperative Study Group on Antihypertensive Agents: Effects of treatment on morbidity in hypertension. I. Results in patients with diastolic blood pressure averaging 115 through 129 mm Hg. *JAMA* 1967;202:1028–1034.

Veterans Administration Cooperative Study Group on Antihypertensive Agents: Effects of treatment on morbidity in hypertension. II. Results in patients with diastolic blood pressure averaging 90 through 114 mm Hg. *JAMA* 1970;213:1143–1152.

Veterans Administration Cooperative Study Group on Antihypertensive Agents: III. Influence of age, diastolic pressure, and prior cardiovascular disease: further analysis of side effects. *Circulation* 1972;45:991–1004.

Veterans Administration Cooperative Study Group on Antihypertensive Agents: Propranolol in the treatment of essential hypertension. *JAMA* 1977;237:2303–2310.

Veterans Administration Cooperative Study Group on Antihypertensive Agents: Comparison of prazosin with hydralazine in patients receiving hydrochlorothiazide. A randomized, double-blind clinical trial. *Circulation* 1981;65:772–779.

Veterans Administration Cooperative Study Group on Antihypertensive Agents: Low-dose captopril for the treatment of mild to moderate hypertension. *Arch Intern Med* 1984;144:1947–1953.

Viberti GC, Bilous RW, Mackintosh D, et al: Long term correction of hyperglycemia and progression of renal failure in insulin dependent diabetes. *Br Med J* 1983;286:589–602.

Virtanen K, Janne J, Frick MH: Response of blood pressure and plasma norepinephrine to propranolol, metoprolol and clonidine during isometric and dynamic exercise. *Eur J Clin Pharmacol* 1982;21:275–279.

Von Holst D: Renal failure as the cause of death in Tupaia belangeri (tree shrews) exposed to persistent social stress. *J Comp Physiol Psychol* 1972;78:236–273.

Waal-Manning HJ, Bolli P: Atenolol vs placebo in mild hypertension: renal, metabolic and stress antipressor effects. *Br J Clin Pharmacol* 1980;9:553–560.

Wada S, Nakayama M, Masaki K: Effects of diltiazem hydrochloride on serum lipids: comparison with beta-blockers. *Clin Ther* 1982;5:163–173.

Waldo R: Prazosin relieves Raynaud's vasospasm. *JAMA* 1979;241:1037.

Walker BA, Deitch MW, Schneider BE, et al: Long-term therapy of hypertension with guanabenz. *Clin Ther* 1981;4:217–228.

Walle T, Conradi EC, Walle UK, et al: The predictable relationship between plasma levels and dose and chronic propranolol therapy. *Clin Pharmacol Ther* 1978;24:668–677.

Weber MA, Drayer JIM: Single agent and combination therapy of essential hypertension. *Am Heart J* 1984;108:311–316.

Weber MA, Zusman RM: Converting enzyme inhibitors in the treatment of hypertension. *Drug Therapy* 1986;16:43–54.

Weber MA, Drayer JIM, Baird WM: Echocardiographic evaluation of left ventricular hypertrophy. *J Cardiovasc Pharmacol* 1986;8:861–869.

Weber MA, Drayer JIM, Kaufman CA: The combined alpha and beta-adrenergic blocker, labetalol, and propranolol in the treatment of high blood pressure: similarities and differences. *J Clin Pharmacol* 1984;24:103–112.

Weber MA, Stokes GS, Gain JM: Comparison of the effects on renin release of beta-adrenergic antagonists with differing properties. *J Clin Invest* 1974;54:1413–1419.

Webster PO, Dyckner T: Diuretic treatment and magnesium losses. *Acta Med Scand Suppl* 1981;647:145–152.

Webster's Third New International Dictionary. Chicago, Encyclopedia Britannica, Inc, 1981.

Weidmann P, Beretta-Piccoli C, Trost BN: Pressor factors and responsiveness in hypertension accompanying diabetes mellitus. *Hypertension* 1985;7:133–142.

Weidmann P, Gerber A, Mordasini R: Effects of antihypertensive therapy on serum lipoproteins. *Hypertension* 1983;5(suppl III):III120–III131.

Weidmann P, Uehlinger DE, Gerber A: Antihypertensive treatment and serum lipoproteins. *J Hypertens* 1985;3:297–306.

Weinberger MH: Comparison of captopril and hydrochlorothiazide alone and in combination in mild to moderate essential hypertension. *Br J Clin Pharmacol* 1982;14(suppl 2):127S–131S.

Weinberger MH: Influence on an angiotensin converting enzyme inhibitor on diuretic-induced metabolic effects in hypertension. *Hypertension* 1983;5(suppl III):III132–III138.

Weinberger MH: Blood pressure and metabolic responses to hydrochlorothiazide, captopril, and the combination in black and white, mild to moderate hypertensive patients. *J Cardiovasc Pharmacol* 1985;7(suppl):S52–S55.

Weinberger MH: Antihypertensive therapy and lipids: paradoxical influences on cardiovascular disease risk. *Am J Med* 1986;80(suppl 2A):64–70.

Weiner BH, Ockene IS, Levine PH, et al: Inhibition of atherosclerosis by cod-liver oil in a hyperlipidemic swine model. *N Engl J Med* 1986;315:841–846.

Weiss YA, Safar ME, London GM, et al: Repeat hemodynamic determinations in borderline hypertension. *Am J Med* 1973;64:382–387.

Wessels F, Hoffmann D, Wagner H, et al: Influence of family history of hypertension on the relationships between blood pressure, body weight, electrolyte metabolism, renin, prolactin and parahormone. *Clin Sci* 1981;61:359–362.

Westaby S, Sapsford RN, Bental H: Return to work and quality of life after surgery for coronary artery disease. *Br Med J* 1979;2:1028–1031.

Westervelt FB, Atuk NO: Methyldopa-induced hypertension (letter). *JAMA* 1974;227:557.

Whang R: Magnesium and potassium interrelationships in cardiac arrhythmias. *Magnesium* 1986;4:127–133.

White AG: Methyldopa and amitriptyline. *Lancet* 1965;2:441–442.

White P: Natural course and prognosis of juvenile diabetes. *Diabetes* 1956;5:455–460.

White WB, Baker LH: Episodic hypertension secondary to panic disorder. *Arch Intern Med* 1986;146:1129–1130.

Whitman HH III, Case DB, Laragh JH, et al: Variable response to oral angiotensin-converting-enzyme blockade in hypertensive scleroderma patients. *Arthritis Rheum* 1982;25:241-248.

Wiley J, Camacho T: Life style and future health: evidence from the Alameda County study. *Prev Med* 1980;9:1–21.

Wilhelmsen L, Svardsudd K, Korsan-Bengtsen K, et al: Fibrinogen as a risk factor for stroke and myocarcial infarction. *N Engl J Med* 1984;311:501–505.

Williams GH: Quality of life and its impact on hypertensive patients. *Am J Med* 1987;82(1):98–103.

Williams GH, Croog SH, Levine S, et al: Impact of antihypertensive therapy on quality of life: effect of hydrochlorothiazide. *J Hypertens* 1987;5(suppl 1):S29–S35.

Williams RR, Dadone MM, Hunt SC, et al: The genetic epidemiology of hypertension: a review of past studies and current results for 948 persons in 48 Utah pedigrees, in Rao DC, Elston RC, Kuller LH et al (eds): *Genetic Epidemiology of Coronary Heart Disease: Past, Present and Future.* New York, Alan R. Liss Inc, 1984, pp 419–442.

Wilson NV, Meyer BM: Early prediction of hypertension using exercise blood pressure. *Prev Med* 1981;10:62–68.

Wilson UW Jr, Untereker W, Hirshfield J: Effects of isosorbide dinitrate and hydralazine on regional metabolic responses to arm exercise in patients with heart failure. *Am J Cardiol* 1981;48:934–938.

Wolfson S, Heinke RA, Herman MV, et al: Propranolol and angina pectoris. *Am J Cardiol* 1966;18:345–353.

Wolthins RA, Froehlicher VF, Fischer J, et al: The response of healthy men to treadmill exercise. *Circulation* 1977;55:153–157.

Wood AJJ, Vestal RE, Branch RA, et al: Age related effects of smoking on elimination of propranolol, antipyrine and indocyanine green (abstract). *Clin Res* 1978;26:297A.

Woods JW, Blythe WB: Management of malignant hypertension complicated by renal insufficiency. *N Engl J Med* 1967;227:57–61.

Yamakado T, Oonishi N, Kondo S, et al: Effects of diltiazem on cardiovascular responses during exercise in systemic hypertension and comparison with propranolol. *Am J Cardiol* 1983;52:1023–1028.

Yorkston NJ, Zaki SA, Themen JF, et al: Safeguards in the treatment of schizophrenia with propranolol. *Postgrad Med J* 1976;52(suppl 4):175–180.

Zanchetti A: Summary of prazosin lipid studies. *Am J Med* 1984;76:122–124.

Zatz R, Dunn BR, Meyer TW, et al: Prevention of diabetic glomerulopathy by pharmacological amelioration of glomerular capillary hypertension. *J Clin Invest* 1986;77:1925–1930.

Zatz R, Meyer TW, Tennke H, et al: Predominance of hemodynamic rather than metabolic factors in the pathogenesis of diabetic glomerulonephropathy. *Proc Nat Acad Sci* 1985;82:5963–5967.

Zubenko GS, Nixon RA: Mood-elevating effect of captopril in depressed patients. *Am J Psychiatry* 1984;141:110–111.

Index

CAUTION: Federal law prohibits dispensing without prescription.

CAPOTEN® TABLETS
Captopril Tablets

DESCRIPTION

CAPOTEN (captopril) is the first of a new class of antihypertensive agents, a specific competitive inhibitor of angiotensin I-converting enzyme (ACE), the enzyme responsible for the conversion of angiotensin I to angiotensin II. Captopril is also effective in the management of heart failure.

CAPOTEN (captopril) is designated chemically as 1-[(2S)-3-mercapto-2-methylpropionyl]-L-proline [MW 217.29] and has the following structure:

Captopril is a white to off-white crystalline powder that may have a slight sulfurous odor; it is soluble in water (approx. 160 mg/mL), methanol, and ethanol and sparingly soluble in chloroform and ethyl acetate.

CAPOTEN (captopril) is available in potencies of 12.5 mg, 25 mg, 50 mg, and 100 mg as scored tablets for oral administration. Inactive ingredients: microcrystalline cellulose, corn starch, lactose, and stearic acid.

CLINICAL PHARMACOLOGY
Mechanism of Action

The mechanism of action of CAPOTEN (captopril) has not yet been fully elucidated. Its beneficial effects in hypertension and heart failure appear to result primarily from suppression of the renin-angiotensin-aldosterone system. However, there is no consistent correlation between renin levels and response to the drug. Renin, an enzyme synthesized by the kidneys, is released into the circulation where it acts on a plasma globulin substrate to produce angiotensin I, a relatively inactive decapeptide. Angiotensin I is then converted by angiotensin converting enzyme (ACE) to angiotensin II, a potent endogenous vasoconstrictor substance. Angiotensin II also stimulates aldosterone secretion from the adrenal cortex, thereby contributing to sodium and fluid retention.

CAPOTEN (captopril) prevents the conversion of angiotensin I to angiotensin II by inhibition of ACE, a peptidyldipeptide carboxy hydrolase. This inhibition has been demonstrated in both healthy human subjects and in animals by showing that the elevation of blood pressure caused by exogenously administered angiotensin I was attenuated or abolished by captopril. In animal studies, captopril did not alter the pressor responses to a number of other agents, including angiotensin II and norepinephrine, indicating specificity of action.

ACE is identical to "bradykininase," and CAPOTEN (captopril) may also interfere with the degradation of the vasodepressor peptide, bradykinin. Increased concentrations of bradykinin or prostaglandin E_2 may also have a role in the therapeutic effect of CAPOTEN.

Inhibition of ACE results in decreased plasma angiotensin II and increased plasma renin activity (PRA), the latter resulting from loss of negative feedback on renin release caused by reduction in angiotensin II. The reduction of angiotensin II leads to decreased aldosterone secretion, and, as a result, small increases in serum potassium may occur along with sodium and fluid loss.

The antihypertensive effects persist for a longer period of time than does demonstrable inhibition of circulating ACE. It is not known whether the ACE present in vascular endothelium is inhibited longer than the ACE in circulating blood.

Pharmacokinetics

After oral administration of therapeutic doses of CAPOTEN (captopril), rapid absorption occurs with peak blood levels at about one hour. The presence of food in the gastrointestinal tract reduces absorption by about 30 to 40 percent; captopril therefore should be given one hour before meals. Based on carbon-14 labeling, average minimal absorption is approximately 75 percent. In a 24-hour period, over 95 percent of the absorbed dose is eliminated in the urine; 40 to 50 percent is unchanged drug; most of the remainder is the disulfide dimer of captopril and captopril-cysteine disulfide.

Approximately 25 to 30 percent of the circulating drug is bound to plasma proteins. The apparent elimination half-life for total radioactivity in blood is probably less than 3 hours. An accurate determination of half-life of unchanged captopril is not, at present, possible, but it is probably less than 2 hours. In patients with renal impairment, however, retention of captopril occurs (see DOSAGE AND ADMINISTRATION).

Pharmacodynamics

Administration of CAPOTEN (captopril) results in a reduction of peripheral arterial resistance in hypertensive patients with either no change, or an increase, in cardiac output. There is an increase in renal blood flow following administration of CAPOTEN (captopril) and glomerular filtration rate is usually unchanged.

Reductions of blood pressure are usually maximal 60 to 90 minutes after oral administration of an individual dose of CAPOTEN (captopril). The duration of effect is dose related. The reduction in blood pressure may be progressive, so to achieve maximal therapeutic effects, several weeks of therapy may be required. The blood pressure lowering effects of captopril and thiazide-type diuretics are additive. In contrast, captopril and beta-blockers have a less than additive effect.

Blood pressure is lowered to about the same extent in both standing and supine positions. Orthostatic effects and tachycardia are infrequent but may occur in volume-depleted patients. Abrupt withdrawal of CAPOTEN has not been associated with a rapid increase in blood pressure.

In patients with heart failure, significantly decreased peripheral (systemic vascular) resistance and blood pressure (afterload), reduced pulmonary capillary wedge pressure (preload) and pulmonary vascular resistance, increased cardiac output, and increased exercise tolerance time (ETT) have been demonstrated. These hemodynamic and clinical effects occur after the first dose and appear to persist for the duration of therapy. Placebo controlled studies of 12 weeks duration show no tolerance to beneficial effects on ETT; open studies, with exposure up to 18 months in some cases, also indicate that ETT benefit is maintained. Clinical improvement has been observed in some patients where acute hemodynamic effects were minimal.

Studies in rats and cats indicate that CAPOTEN (captopril) does not cross the blood-brain barrier to any significant extent.

INDICATIONS AND USAGE

Hypertension: CAPOTEN (captopril) is indicated for the treatment of hypertension.

In using CAPOTEN, consideration should be given to the risk of neutropenia/agranulocytosis (see WARNINGS).

CAPOTEN may be used as initial therapy for patients with normal renal function, in whom the risk is relatively low. In patients with impaired renal function, particularly those with collagen vascular disease, captopril should be reserved for hypertensives who have either developed unacceptable side effects on other drugs, or have failed to respond satisfactorily to drug combinations.

CAPOTEN is effective alone and in combination with other antihypertensive agents, especially thiazide-type diuretics. The blood pressure lowering effects of captopril and thiazides are approximately additive.

Heart Failure: CAPOTEN (captopril) is indicated in patients with heart failure who have not responded adequately to or cannot be controlled by conventional diuretic and digitalis therapy. CAPOTEN is to be used with diuretics and digitalis.

CONTRAINDICATIONS

CAPOTEN is contraindicated in patients who are hypersensitive to this product.

WARNINGS

Neutropenia/Agranulocytosis

Neutropenia (< 1000/mm³) with myeloid hypoplasia has resulted from use of captopril. About half of the neutropenic patients developed systemic or oral cavity infections or other features of the syndrome of agranulocytosis.

The risk of neutropenia is dependent on the clinical status of the patient:

In clinical trials in patients with hypertension who have normal renal function (serum creatinine less than 1.6 mg/dL and no collagen vascular disease), neutropenia has been seen in one patient out of over 8,600 exposed.

In patients with some degree of renal failure (serum creatinine at least 1.6 mg/dL) but no collagen vascular disease, the risk of neutropenia in clinical trials was about 1 per 500, a frequency over 15 times that for uncomplicated hypertension. Daily doses of captopril were relatively high in these patients, particularly in view of their diminished renal function. In foreign marketing experience in patients with renal failure, use of allopurinol concomitantly with captopril has been associated with neutropenia but this association has not appeared in U.S. reports.

In patients with collagen vascular diseases (e.g., systemic lupus erythematosus, scleroderma) and impaired renal function, neutropenia occurred in 3.7 percent of patients in clinical trials.

While none of the over 750 patients in formal clinical trials of heart failure developed neutropenia, it has occurred during the subsequent clinical experience. About half of the reported cases had serum creatinine ≥ 1.6 mg/dL and more than 75 percent were in patients also receiving procainamide. In heart failure, it appears that the same risk factors for neutropenia are present.

The neutropenia has usually been detected within three months after captopril was started. Bone marrow examinations in patients with neutropenia consistently showed myeloid hypoplasia, frequently accompanied by erythroid hypoplasia and decreased numbers of megakaryocytes (e.g., hypoplastic bone marrow and pancytopenia); anemia and thrombocytopenia were sometimes seen.

In general, neutrophils returned to normal in about two weeks after captopril was discontinued, and serious infections were limited to clinically complex patients. About 13 percent of the cases of neutropenia have ended fatally, but almost all fatalities were in patients with serious illness, having collagen vascular disease, renal failure, heart failure or immunosuppressant therapy, or a combination of these complicating factors.

Evaluation of the hypertensive or heart failure patient should always include assessment of renal function.

If captopril is used in patients with impaired renal function, white blood cell and differential counts should be evaluated prior to starting treatment and at approximately two-week intervals for about three months, then periodically.

In patients with collagen vascular disease or who are exposed to other drugs known to affect the white cells or immune response, particularly when there is impaired renal function, captopril should be used only after an assessment of benefit and risk, and then with caution.

All patients treated with captopril should be told to report any signs of infection (e.g., sore throat, fever). If infection is suspected, white cell counts should be performed without delay.

Since discontinuation of captopril and other drugs has generally led to prompt return of the white count to normal, upon confirmation of neutropenia (neutrophil count < 1000/mm³) the physician should withdraw captopril and closely follow the patient's course.

Proteinuria

Total urinary proteins greater than 1 g per day were seen in about 0.7 percent of patients receiving captopril. About 90 percent of affected patients had evidence of prior renal disease or received relatively high doses of captopril (in excess of 150 mg/day), or both. The nephrotic syndrome occurred in about one-fifth of proteinuric patients. In most cases, proteinuria subsided or cleared within six months whether or not captopril was continued. Parameters of renal function, such as BUN and creatinine, were seldom altered in the patients with proteinuria.

Since most cases of proteinuria occurred by the eighth month of therapy with captopril, patients with prior renal disease or those receiving captopril at doses greater than 150 mg per day, should have urinary protein estimations (dip-stick on first morning urine) prior to treatment, and periodically thereafter.

Hypotension

Excessive hypotension was rarely seen in hypertensive patients but is a possible consequence of captopril use in severely salt/volume depleted persons such as those treated vigorously with diuretics, for example, patients with severe congestive heart failure (see PRECAUTIONS [Drug Interactions]).

In heart failure, where the blood pressure was either normal or low, transient decreases in mean blood pressure greater than 20 percent were recorded in about half of the patients. This transient hypotension may occur after any of the first several doses and is usually well tolerated, producing either no symptoms or brief mild lightheadedness, although in rare instances it has been associated with arrhythmia or conduction defects. Hypotension was the reason for discontinuation of drug in 3.6 percent of patients with heart failure.

BECAUSE OF THE POTENTIAL FALL IN BLOOD PRESSURE IN THESE PATIENTS, THERAPY SHOULD BE STARTED UNDER VERY CLOSE MEDICAL SUPERVISION. A starting dose of 6.25 or 12.5 mg tid may minimize the hypotensive effect. Patients should be followed closely for the first two weeks of treatment and whenever the dose of captopril and/or diuretic is increased.

Hypotension is not *per se* a reason to discontinue captopril. Some decrease of systemic blood pressure is a common and desirable observation upon initiation of CAPOTEN (captopril) treatment in heart failure. The magnitude of the decrease is greatest early in the course of treatment; this effect stabilizes within a week or two, and generally returns to pretreatment levels, without a decrease in therapeutic efficacy, within two months.

PRECAUTIONS

General

Impaired Renal Function

Hypertension—Some patients with renal disease, particularly those with severe renal artery stenosis, have developed increases in BUN and serum creatinine after reduction of blood pressure with captopril. Captopril dosage reduction and/or discontinuation of diuretic may be required. For some of these patients, it may not be possible to normalize blood pressure and maintain adequate renal perfusion.

Heart Failure—About 20 percent of patients develop stable elevations of BUN and serum creatinine greater than 20 percent above normal or baseline upon long-term treatment with captopril. Less than 5 percent of patients, generally those with severe preexisting renal disease, required discontinuation of treatment due to progressively increasing creatinine; subsequent improvement probably depends upon the severity of the underlying renal disease.

See CLINICAL PHARMACOLOGY, DOSAGE AND ADMINISTRATION, ADVERSE REACTIONS [Altered Laboratory Findings].

Valvular Stenosis: There is concern, on theoretical grounds, that patients with aortic stenosis might be at particular risk of decreased coronary perfusion when treated with vasodilators because they do not develop as much afterload reduction as others.

Surgery/Anesthesia: In patients undergoing major surgery or during anesthesia with agents that produce hypotension, captopril will block angiotensin II formation secondary to compensatory renin release. If hypotension occurs and is considered to be due to this mechanism, it can be corrected by volume expansion.

Information for Patients

Patients should be told to report promptly any indication of infection (e.g., sore throat, fever), which may be a sign of neutropenia, or of progressive edema which might be related to proteinuria and nephrotic syndrome.

All patients should be cautioned that excessive perspiration and dehydration may lead to an excessive fall in blood pressure because of reduction in fluid volume. Other causes of volume depletion such as vomiting or diarrhea may also lead to a fall in blood pressure; patients should be advised to consult with the physician.

Patients should be warned against interruption or discontinuation of medication unless instructed by the physician.

Heart failure patients on captopril therapy should be cautioned against rapid increases in physical activity.

Patients should be informed that CAPOTEN (captopril) should be taken one hour before meals (see DOSAGE AND ADMINISTRATION).

Drug Interactions

Hypotension—Patients on Diuretic Therapy: Patients on diuretics and especially those in whom diuretic therapy was recently instituted, as well as those on severe dietary salt restriction or dialysis, may occasionally experience a precipitous reduction of blood pressure usually within the first hour after receiving the initial dose of captopril.

The possibility of hypotensive effects with captopril can be minimized by either discontinuing the diuretic or increasing the salt intake approximately one week prior to initiation of treatment with CAPOTEN (captopril) or initiating therapy with small doses (6.25 or 12.5 mg). Alternatively, provide medical supervision for at least one hour after the initial dose. If hypotension occurs, the patient should be placed in a supine position and, if necessary, receive an intravenous infusion of normal saline. This transient hypotensive response is not a contraindication to further doses which can be given without difficulty once the blood pressure has increased after volume expansion.

Agents Having Vasodilator Activity: Data on the effect of concomitant use of other vasodilators in patients receiving CAPOTEN for heart failure are not available; therefore, nitroglycerin or other nitrates (as used for management of angina) or other drugs having vasodilator activity should, if possible, be discontinued before starting CAPOTEN. If resumed during CAPOTEN therapy, such agents should be administered cautiously, and perhaps at lower dosage.

Agents Causing Renin Release: Captopril's effect will be augmented by antihypertensive agents that cause renin release. For example, diuretics (e.g., thiazides) may activate the renin-angiotensin-aldosterone system.

Agents Affecting Sympathetic Activity: The sympathetic nervous system may be especially important in supporting blood pressure in patients receiving captopril alone or with diuretics. Therefore, agents affecting sympathetic activity (e.g., ganglionic blocking agents or adrenergic neuron blocking agents) should be used with caution. Beta-adrenergic blocking drugs add some further antihypertensive effect to captopril, but the overall response is less than additive.

Agents Increasing Serum Potassium: Since captopril decreases aldosterone production, elevation of serum potassium may occur. Potassium-sparing diuretics such as spironolactone, triamterene, or amiloride, or potassium supplements should be given only for documented hypokalemia, and then with caution, since they may lead to a significant increase of serum potassium. Salt substitutes containing potassium should also be used with caution.

Inhibitors Of Endogenous Prostaglandin Synthesis: It has been reported that indomethacin may reduce the antihypertensive effect of captopril, especially in cases of low renin hypertension. Other nonsteroidal anti-inflammatory agents (e.g., aspirin) may also have this effect.

Drug/Laboratory Test Interaction

Captopril may cause a false-positive urine test for acetone.

Carcinogenesis, Mutagenesis and Impairment of Fertility

Two-year studies with doses of 50 to 1350 mg/kg/day in mice and rats failed to show any evidence of carcinogenic potential.

Studies in rats have revealed no impairment of fertility.

Animal Toxicology

Chronic oral toxicity studies were conducted in rats (2 years), dogs (47 weeks; 1 year), mice (2 years), and monkeys (1 year). Significant drug-related toxicity included effects on hematopoiesis, renal toxicity, erosion/ulceration of the stomach, and variation of retinal blood vessels.

Reductions in hemoglobin and/or hematocrit values were seen in mice, rats, and monkeys at doses 50 to 150 times the maximum recommended human dose (MRHD). Anemia, leukopenia, thrombocytopenia, and bone marrow suppression occurred in dogs at doses 8 to 30 times MRHD. The reductions in hemoglobin and hematocrit values in rats and mice were only significant at 1 year and returned to normal with continued dosing by the end of the study. Marked anemia was seen at all dose levels (8 to 30 times MRHD) in dogs, whereas moderate to marked leukopenia was noted only at 15 and 30 times MRHD and thrombocytopenia at 30 times MRHD. The anemia could be reversed upon discontinuation of dosing. Bone marrow suppression occurred to a varying degree, being associated only with dogs that died or were sacrificed in a moribund condition in the 1 year study. However, in the 47-week study at a dose 30 times MRHD, bone marrow suppression was found to be reversible upon continued drug administration.

Captopril caused hyperplasia of the juxtaglomerular apparatus of the kidneys at doses 7 to 200 times the MRHD in rats and mice, at 20 to 60 times MRHD in monkeys, and at 30 times the MRHD in dogs.

Gastric erosions/ulcerations were increased in incidence at 20 and 200 times MRHD in male rats and at 30 and 65 times MRHD in dogs and monkeys, respectively. Rabbits developed gastric and intestinal ulcers when given oral doses approximately 30 times MRHD for only 5 to 7 days.

In the two-year rat study, irreversible and progressive variations in the caliber of retinal vessels (focal sacculations and constrictions) occurred at all dose levels (7 to 200 times MRHD) in a dose-related fashion. The effect was first observed in the 88th week of dosing, with a progressively increased incidence thereafter, even after cessation of dosing.

Pregnancy: Category C

Captopril was embryocidal in rabbits when given in doses about 2 to 70 times (on a mg/kg basis) the maximum recommended human dose, and low incidences of craniofacial malformations were seen. These effects in rabbits were most probably due to the particularly marked decrease in blood pressure caused by the drug in this species.

Captopril given to pregnant rats at 400 times the recommended human dose continuously during gestation and lactation caused a reduction in neonatal survival.

No teratogenic effects (malformations) have been observed after large doses of captopril in hamsters and rats.

Captopril crosses the human placenta.

There are no adequate and well-controlled studies in pregnant women. Captopril should be used during pregnancy, or for patients likely to become pregnant, only if the potential benefit justifies a potential risk to the fetus.

Nursing Mothers

Concentrations of captopril in human milk are approximately one percent of those in maternal blood. The effect of low levels of captopril on the nursing infant has not been determined. Caution should be exercised when captopril is administered to a nursing woman, and, in general, nursing should be interrupted.

Pediatric Use

Safety and effectiveness in children have not been established although there is limited experience with the use of captopril in children from 2 months to 15 years of age with secondary hypertension and varying degrees of renal insufficiency. Dosage, on a weight basis, was comparable to that used in adults. CAPOTEN (captopril) should be used in children only if other measures for controlling blood pressure have not been effective.

ADVERSE REACTIONS

Reported incidences are based on clinical trials involving approximately 7000 patients.

Renal—About one of 100 patients developed proteinuria (see WARNINGS).

Each of the following has been reported in approximately 1 to 2 of 1000 patients and are of uncertain relationship to drug use: renal insufficiency, renal failure, polyuria, oliguria, and urinary frequency.

Hematologic—Neutropenia/agranulocytosis has occurred (see WARNINGS). Cases of anemia, thrombocytopenia, and pancytopenia have been reported.

Dermatologic—Rash, often with pruritus, and sometimes with fever, arthralgia, and eosinophilia, occurred in about 4 to 7 (depending on renal status and dose) of 100 patients, usually during the first four weeks of therapy. It is usually maculopapular, and rarely urticarial. The rash is usually mild and disappears within a few days of dosage reduction, short-term treatment with an antihistaminic agent, and/or discontinuing therapy; remission may occur even if captopril is continued.

Pruritus, without rash, occurs in about 2 of 100 patients. Between 7 and 10 percent of patients with skin rash have shown an eosinophilia and/or positive ANA titers. A reversible associated pemphigoid-like lesion, and photosensitivity, have also been reported.

Angioedema of the face, mucous membranes of the mouth, or of the extremities has been observed in approximately 1 of 1000 patients and is reversible on discontinuance of captopril therapy. One case of laryngeal edema has been reported.

Flushing or pallor has been reported in 2 to 5 of 1000 patients.

Cardiovascular—Hypotension may occur; see WARNINGS and PRECAUTIONS [Drug Interactions] for discussion of hypotension on initiation of captopril therapy.

Tachycardia, chest pain, and palpitations have each been observed in approximately 1 of 100 patients.

Angina pectoris, myocardial infarction, Raynaud's syndrome, and congestive heart failure have each occurred in 2 to 3 of 1000 patients.

Dysgeusia—Approximately 2 to 4 (depending on renal status and dose) of 100 patients developed a diminution or loss of taste perception. Taste impairment is reversible and usually self-limited (2 to 3 months) even with continued drug administration. Weight loss may be associated with the loss of taste.

The following have been reported in about 0.5 to 2 percent of patients but did not appear at increased frequency compared to placebo or other treatments used in controlled trials: gastric irritation, abdominal pain, nausea, vomiting, diarrhea, anorexia, constipation, aphthous ulcers, peptic ulcer, dizziness, headache, malaise, fatigue, insomnia, dry mouth, dyspnea, cough, alopecia, paresthesias.

Altered Laboratory Findings
Elevations of liver enzymes have been noted in a few patients but no causal relationship to captopril use has been established. Rare cases of cholestatic jaundice, and of hepatocellular injury with or without secondary cholestasis, have been reported in association with captopril administration.

A transient elevation of BUN and serum creatinine may occur, especially in patients who are volume-depleted or who have renovascular hypertension. In instances of rapid reduction of longstanding or severely elevated blood pressure, the glomerular filtration rate may decrease transiently, also resulting in transient rises in serum creatinine and BUN.

Small increases in the serum potassium concentration frequently occur, especially in patients with renal impairment (see PRECAUTIONS).

OVERDOSAGE
Correction of hypotension would be of primary concern. Volume expansion with an intravenous infusion of normal saline is the treatment of choice for restoration of blood pressure.

Captopril may be removed from the general circulation by hemodialysis.

DOSAGE AND ADMINISTRATION
CAPOTEN (captopril) should be taken one hour before meals. Dosage must be individualized.

Hypertension—Initiation of therapy requires consideration of recent antihypertensive drug treatment, the extent of blood pressure elevation, salt restriction, and other clinical circumstances. If possible, discontinue the patient's previous antihypertensive drug regimen for one week before starting CAPOTEN.

The initial dose of CAPOTEN (captopril) is 25 mg bid or tid. If satisfactory reduction of blood pressure has not been achieved after one or two weeks, the dose may be increased to 50 mg bid or tid. Concomitant sodium restriction may be beneficial when CAPOTEN is used alone.

The dose of CAPOTEN in hypertension usually does not exceed 50 mg tid. Therefore, if the blood pressure has not been satisfactorily controlled after one to two weeks at this dose, (and the patient is not already receiving a diuretic), a modest dose of a thiazide-type diuretic (e.g., hydrochlorothiazide, 25 mg daily), should be added. The diuretic dose may be increased at one- to two-week intervals until its highest usual antihypertensive dose is reached.

If CAPOTEN is being started in a patient already receiving a diuretic, CAPOTEN therapy should be initiated under close medical supervision (see WARNINGS and PRECAUTIONS [Drug Interactions] regarding hypotension), with dosage and titration of CAPOTEN as noted above.

If further blood pressure reduction is required, the dose of CAPOTEN may be increased to 100 mg bid or tid and then, if necessary, to 150 mg bid or tid (while continuing the diuretic). The usual dose range is 25 to 150 mg bid or tid. A maximum daily dose of 450 mg CAPOTEN should not be exceeded.

For patients with severe hypertension (e.g., accelerated or malignant hypertension), when temporary discontinuation of current antihypertensive therapy is not practical or desirable, or when prompt titration to more normotensive blood pressure levels is indicated, diuretic should be continued but other current antihypertensive medication stopped and CAPOTEN dosage promptly initiated at 25 mg bid or tid, under close medical supervision.

When necessitated by the patient's clinical condition, the daily dose of CAPOTEN may be increased every 24 hours or less under continuous medical supervision until a satisfactory blood pressure response is obtained or the maximum dose of CAPOTEN is reached. In this regimen, addition of a more potent diuretic, e.g., furosemide, may also be indicated.

Beta-blockers may also be used in conjunction with CAPOTEN therapy (see PRECAUTIONS [Drug Interactions]), but the effects of the two drugs are less than additive.

Heart Failure—Initiation of therapy requires consideration of recent diuretic therapy and the possibility of severe salt/volume depletion. In patients with either normal or low blood pressure, who have been vigorously treated with diuretics and who may be hyponatremic and/or hypovolemic, a starting dose of 6.25 or 12.5 mg tid may minimize the magnitude or duration of the hypotensive effect (see WARNINGS, [Hypotension]); for these patients, titration to the usual daily dosage can then occur within the next several days.

For most patients the usual initial daily dosage is 25 mg tid. After a dose of 50 mg tid is reached, further increases in dosage should be delayed, where possible, for at least two weeks to determine if a satisfactory response occurs. Most patients studied have had a satisfactory clinical improvement at 50 or 100 mg tid. A maximum daily dose of 450 mg of CAPOTEN (captopril) should not be exceeded.

CAPOTEN is to be used in conjunction with a diuretic and digitalis. CAPOTEN therapy must be initiated under very close medical supervision.

Dosage Adjustment in Renal Impairment—Because CAPOTEN (captopril) is excreted primarily by the kidneys, excretion rates are reduced in patients with impaired renal function. These patients will take longer to reach steady-state captopril levels and will reach higher steady-state levels for a given daily dose than patients with normal renal function. Therefore, these patients may respond to smaller or less frequent doses.

Accordingly, for patients with significant renal impairment, initial daily dosage of CAPOTEN (captopril) should be reduced, and smaller increments utilized for titration, which should be quite slow (one- to two-week intervals). After the desired therapeutic effect has been achieved, the dose should be slowly back-titrated to determine the minimal effective dose. When concomitant diuretic therapy is required, a loop diuretic (e.g., furosemide), rather than a thiazide diuretic, is preferred in patients with severe renal impairment.

HOW SUPPLIED
12.5 mg tablets in bottles of 100 (NDC 0003-0450-54), **25 mg tablets** in bottles of 100 (NDC 0003-0452-50) and 1000 (NDC 0003-0452-75), **50 mg tablets** in bottles of 100 (NDC 0003-0482-50) and 1000 (NDC 0003-0482-75), and **100 mg tablets** in bottles of 100 (NDC 0003-0485-50). Bottles contain a desiccant-charcoal canister.

Unimatic® unit-dose packs containing 100 tablets are also available for each potency: **12.5 mg** (NDC 0003-0450-51), **25 mg** (NDC 0003-0452-51), **50 mg** (NDC 0003-0482-51), and **100 mg** (NDC 0003-0485-51).

The **12.5 mg tablet** is a flat oval with a partial bisect bar; the **25 mg tablet** is a biconvex rounded square with a quadrisect bar; the **50 and 100 mg tablets** are biconvex ovals with a bisect bar.

All captopril tablets are white and may exhibit a slight sulfurous odor. Tablet identification numbers: **12.5 mg**, 450; **25 mg**, 452; **50 mg**, 482; and **100 mg**, 485.

Storage
Do not store above 86° F. Keep bottles tightly closed (protect from moisture).

E. R. Squibb & Sons, Inc.
Princeton, NJ 08540